Diver Medic

Student Manual and Handouts

Commander Ronald L. Ellerman (ret.)

No part of this book may be reproduced, transmitted, or stored in any form or by any means electronic or mechanical, including photocopying, recording, scanning, digitizing, or by any information storage or retrieval system, without the expressed written consent of the author.

Diver Medic Student Handouts

By Ronald L. Ellerman

© Copyright 2018 by Ronald L. Ellerman. All Rights Reserved

Cover Design: Ronald L. Ellerman

Disclaimer

This textbook is intended to be utilized in the teaching of a medical course by qualified and knowledgeable instructors in the procedures and treatments contained herein. It is not intended to be utilized as a self-study or self-taught guide.

The procedures and protocols in this textbook are based on the most current recommendations and practices of responsible medical sources. Hyperbaric Training Associates, the author, and the publisher, however, make no guarantee as to, and assume no responsibility for, the correctness, sufficiency, or completeness of such information or recommendations. Other or additional safety and medical measures may be required under particular circumstances. The medical field is extremely dynamic with regards to new procedures and equipment. Readers are encouraged and advised to check the most current information provided, on procedures featured, and by the manufacturer of each product featured. To the fullest extent of the law, neither Hyperbaric Training Associates, the author, nor the publisher assumes any liability for any injury and/or damage to persons or property arising out of or related to any use of the material contained in this textbook.

This textbook is intended solely as a guide to the appropriate measures and procedures to be utilized and employed when rendering emergency care to the sick and injured. It is not intended as a statement of the standard of care required in any particular situation or circumstance, due to the fact that circumstances and patient conditions may vary widely from one emergency to another. Nor is it intended that this textbook should, in any way, advise emergency medical personnel concerning legal authority to perform the activities and procedures discussed herein. Such determination shall be made locally and with the aid of legal counsel only.

Users of this textbook are further warned that the use of any technique, procedure, treatment, drug, or other substance must be authorized by their medical control and direction through standing orders, protocols, or online consultation and direction and must also, where appropriate, be in accordance with local, state, federal, and international laws and regulations.

Gender Statement

The English language has historically given preference to the male gender. In many cases, the pronouns, he and his, are commonly used to describe both genders. Since the male pronouns still dominate our speech and language, they have been used throughout this textbook to portray both male and female diver medics and patients for brevity. The author realizes and acknowledges that female divers and diver medics play an important and indispensable role in this industry and this usage in no way diminishes their importance.

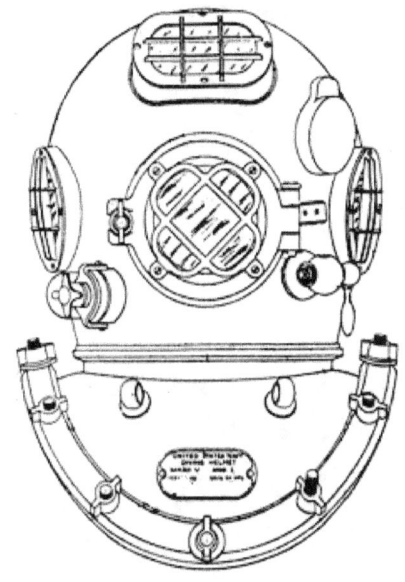

Hyperbaric Training Associates

Standards & Procedures of Practical Skills Manual

July 2018

www.divermedicaltechnician.com

This manual is intended to provide examples of tried and proven techniques of caring for patients with the various injuries or illnesses that EMS personnel will encounter in the field. It does not provide the only method or technique that may be an acceptable approach in caring for an injury or illness. However, since the various certification examinations used are based on the current edition of this document as well as the current edition of the US DOT National Standard Curriculum, it is an advantage to use these skill procedures as the basis for practice. This is a consensus document, endorsed by EMS Training Centers and regional and local physician medical direction who are charged with developing and promulgating minimum standards of care for EMS providers

This manual contains descriptions of those skills included in the scope of practice for all EMS personnel. The scope of practice for each level of provider, as defined by the Diving Medical Officer and local protocol, shall define which of these skills may be used at each provider level.

Table of Contents

SECTION 1 – ASSESSMENT TOOLS: BLOOD PRESSURE MEASUREMENT; PULSE OXIMITY; BLOOD GLUCOSE MEASUREMENT; 12-LEAD ECG; CAPNOGRAPHY 9
    I. BLOOD PRESSURE MEASUREMENT 9
    II. PULSE OXIMITY 10
    III. BLOOD GLUCOSE MEASUREMENT 10
    IV. 12-LEAD ECG 11
    V. END TITAL CO2 (WAVEFORM CAPNOGRAPHY) 12

SECTION 2 – LIFTING AND MOVING PATIENTS 13
    III. NON-URGENT MOVES: 14
    IV. EQUIPMENT MOVES: 16

SECTION 3 – AIRWAY AND RESPIRATORY MANAGEMENT 17
    I. OXYGEN ADMINISTRATION / DISCONTINUANCE 17
    II. PATIENT POSITIONING (Non-trauma unresponsive patient) 18
    III. OROPHARYNGEAL AIRWAY INSERTION (Unresponsive patient with no gag reflex) 18
    IV. NASOPHARYNGEAL AIRWAY INSERTION (Responsive or unresponsive patient) 19
    V. NON-VISUALIZED ADVANCED AIRWAY INSERTION 19
    VI. ENDOTRACHEAL TUBE INSERTION AND REMOVAL 23
    VII. PHARYNGEAL AND TRACHEOBRONCHIAL SUCTIONING 27
    VIII. LARYNGOSCOPE AND MAGILL FORCEPS 28
    IX. BAG-VALVE-MASK (BVM) 29
    X. MANUALLY TRIGGERED VENTILATION DEVICES 29
    XI. POCKET MASK 30
    XII. CONTINUOUS POSITIVE AIR PRESSURE 30
    XIII. PERCUTANEOUS SURGICAL / NEEDLE CRICOTHYROTOMY 31

SECTION 4 – PATIENT ASSESSMENT 34
    I. PATIENT ASSESSMENT 34

SECTION 5 – CARDIAC MANAGEMENT 38
    I. CARDIOPULMONARY RESUSCITATION 38
    II. AUTOMATED EXTERNAL DEFIBRILLATION 38
    III. ELECTRICAL THERAPY 38
    IV. CARDIAC MONITORING 42

SECTION 6 – MEDICATION PREPARATION AND ADMINISTRATION 43
    I. ENTERAL ROUTES: ORAL, SUBLINGUAL, BUCCAL, GASTRIC TUBE, AND RECTAL MEDICATIONS 43

II.	INHALED MEDICATIONS	45
III.	TOPICAL MEDICATIONS	47
IV.	INJECTABLE MEDICATIONS	48
V.	INTRAVENOUS / INTRAOSSEOUS ADMINISTRATION AND CARE	52

SECTION 7 – MANAGEMENT OF SOFT TISSUE INJURIES 59
    I. BLEEDING CONTROL 59
    II. HEAD 60
    III. EYE 60
    IV. NECK 61
    V. TORSO 61
    VI. EXTREMITIES 63
    VII. BURNS 64

SECTION 8 – PNEUMATIC ANTI-SHOCK GARMENT 66

SECTION 9 – ORTHOPEDIC TRAUMA 68
    I. THORAX 68
    II. EXTREMITIES 69

SECTION 10 – SPINAL INJURIES 74

SECTION 11 – OTHER ADVANCED LIFE SUPPORT SKILLS 83
    I. NASOGASTRIC / OROGASTRIC TUBE INSERTION 83
    II. THORACENTESIS 84

PRACTICAL SKILLS SHEETS AND PRACTICE WRIITEN EXAMINATION 85

TENDER BAILOUT TABLE FOR OXYGEN TREATMENT TABLES 121

U.S.NAVY NEUROLOGICAL EXAMINATION (REVISION 7) 139

SECTION 1 – ASSESSMENT TOOLS: BLOOD PRESSURE MEASUREMENT; PULSE OXIMITY; BLOOD GLUCOSE MEASUREMENT; 12-LEAD ECG; CAPNOGRAPHY

- OBJECTIVES:
- To consistently obtain accurate blood pressure measurement through the use of auscultation and palpation methods, and use of mechanical units.
- To accurately measure the percent of circulating hemoglobin saturated with oxygen.
- To accurately measure the blood glucose level through the use of a glucometer
- To acquire and transmit a 12-lead ECG.
- To objectively measure the partial pressure of End-tidal CO2.

I. BLOOD PRESSURE MEASUREMENT

POINTS OF EMPHASIS:
- Correctly size the blood pressure cuff
- The inflatable portion of the cuff's length should encircle at least 80 percent of the upper arm and should be wide enough to cover 40 percent of the arm at mid-point of the bladder.
- A cuff that is too large will give a false low reading.
- A cuff that is too small will give a false high reading.
- Locate the brachial pulse in the antecubital space.
- Inflate the cuff 30 mmHg above the point at which the pulse is lost.
- Deflate the cuff proportionate to the rate of the pulse and record the results.

SKILLS:
A. PALPATION METHOD
   1. Position the patient with the arm at heart level.
   2. Palpate the brachial or radial pulse.
   3. Apply the cuff snugly around the extremity with the lower edge at least one inch above the antecubital space with the cuff's bladder centered over the brachial artery.
   4. Inflate the blood pressure cuff to 30 mmHg above the point at which the pulse disappears.
   5. Deflate the cuff slowly while noting the point at which the pulse is felt to return.
   6. Record the systolic blood pressure as #/P.

B. AUSCULTATORY METHOD
   1. Position the patient with the arm at heart level.
   2. Palpate the brachial pulse.
   3. Apply the cuff snugly around the extremity with the lower edge at least one inch from the antecubital space and the cuff's bladder centered over the brachial artery.
   4. Insert the stethoscope earpieces in ears with earpieces pointing slightly forward; test the diaphragm for sound conduction by gently tapping on diaphragm.
   5. Palpate or auscultate the brachial artery while inflating the cuff to 30mmHg above the loss of pulse.
   6. Deflate slowly with stethoscope diaphragm over the brachial artery listening for the return of the pulse and then the disappearance of the pulse.
      - The point of pulse return is the systolic pressure
      - The point of disappearance is the diastolic pressure

C. AUTOMATIC BLOOD PRESSURE MEASURING DEVICES
   1. Various types of equipment available
   2. Follow manufacturers recommendations

II. PULSE OXIMITY

POINTS OF EMPHASIS
- Do not depend on oximeter reading alone to assess the patient's oxygenation status.
- Typically, a normal pulse oximetry reading is greater than 93%. For some chronically ill patients, the percentage may be lower.
- The accuracy of the measurement may be affected by low blood flow, CO poisoning, nail polish, gel nails, dirt, jaundice, patient movement, bright light, and hypothermia. If the pulse count or waveform does not correlate with the patient's pulse, the accuracy of the reading should be questioned. Care should be directed by other signs and symptoms of the patient.
- A pediatric adhesive style transducer can be utilized for an adult patient when the finger does not provide a reading. Adhere the transducer over the bridge of the patient's nose.

SKILLS:
A. STANDARD METHOD
   1. Select and place the appropriate transducer on the patient (finger, toe, earlobe, etc.)
      - Clean the site with an alcohol swab if necessary.
      - Tape around the great toe or foot – pediatric patient
      - Tape across the bridge of the patient's nose – pediatric transducer on adult patient.
   2. Turn on the monitor
   3. Verify that pulse reading on the oximeter is equal to the patient's pulse.
   4. Note and record the reading.

III. BLOOD GLUCOSE MEASUREMENT

POINTS OF EMPHASIS
- Record reading in mg/dl.
- Consider all patients with altered level of consciousness.
- Ensure that the unit is calibrated per manufactures specifications.
- Check expiration date of the test strips.
- Protocols may suggest wiping away the first drop of blood, using the second for the sample.

SKILLS:
A. EMR Blood Glucose Monitoring with specific training and approvals in accordance with DMO approved protocols.
   1. Prepare equipment (glucometer, lancet device, alcohol wipes, Band-Aid®, gauze pad, and sharps container) in advance, according to manufacturer's recommendations.
   2. Clean finger with alcohol prep pad, allowing alcohol to dry for 30 seconds
   3. Turn unit on
   4. Confirm test strip code with glucometer display reading
   5. Prick finger with lancet to obtain blood sample
   6. Apply sample to test strip
   7. Cover puncture site with Band-Aid if bleeding continues
   8. Properly dispose of lancet

B. Note and record reading

IV. 12-LEAD ECG

POINTS OF EMPHASIS:
- Identify need for 12-lead ECG
- Cover exposed areas as appropriate.
- If transporting, stop the vehicle or vessel, if possible, in order to acquire an accurate ECG.

SKILLS:
A. Prepare the skin if needed.
B. Place the patient in a recumbent position.
C. Connect the electrodes to the cable
D. Apply the electrodes to the limbs (the limb leads must be placed distal to the shoulders and distal to the hip joints to obtain an accurate ECG)
   1. LL=Left leg
   2. RL=Right leg
   3. LA=Left arm
   4. RA=Right arm
E. Place chest leads using appropriate landmarks (see 12-lead placement figure)
   1. V1 = 4th intercostal space just to the right of the sternum (1)
   2. V2 = 4th intercostal space just to the left of the sternum (2)
   3. V3 = halfway between V2 and V4 (3)
   4. V4 = 5th intercostal space in the mid-clavicular line (4)
   5. V5 = anterior axillary line, level with V4 (5)
   6. V6 = mid-axillary line level with V4 (6)
F. Enter patient information into monitor.
G. Instruct the patient to remain still and quiet while acquiring tracing
H. Acquire the 12-Lead ECG tracing.
I. Check 12-Lead for quality
J. Transmit electronically or print tracings from monitor.

PLACEMENT OF 12-LEAD ELECTRODES

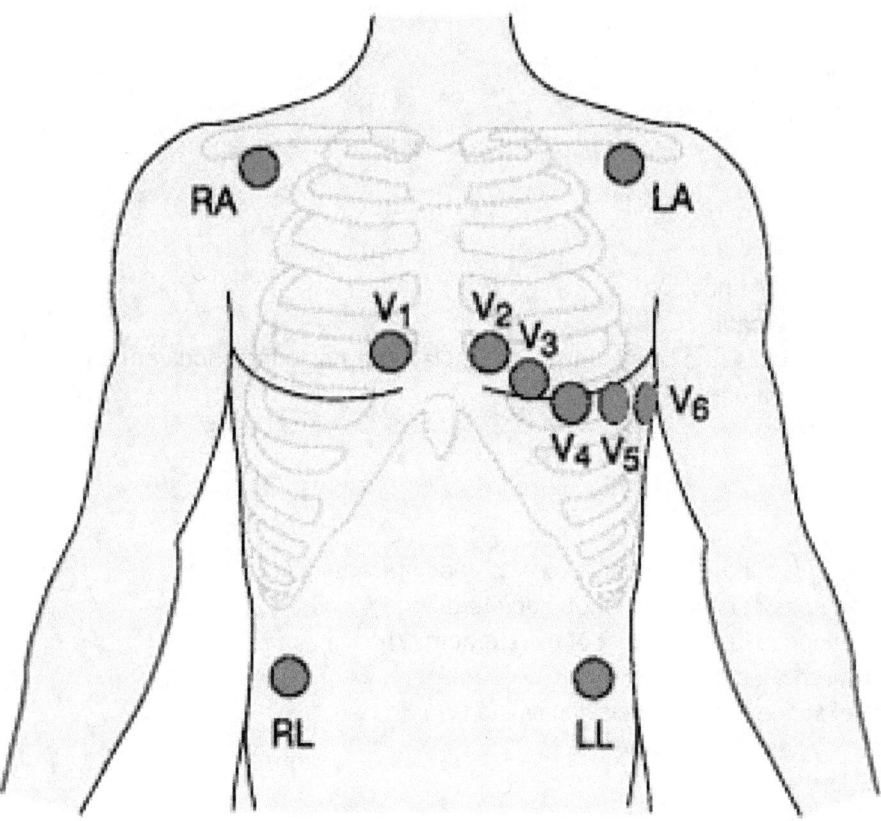

V. END TITAL CO2 (WAVEFORM CAPNOGRAPHY)

POINTS OF EMPHASIS:
- Identify the need for End-tidal CO2 monitoring.
- Monitors the measurement of carbon dioxide in the airway at the end of each breath. Helps determine ventilation, circulation, and cellular perfusion.
- Displayed as a numeric value and/or graphic waveform.
- Prepare equipment according to the manufacturers recommendation.
- Normal values = 35-45 mmHg
- Excess secretions or blood can interfere with the sensors ability to read the EtCO2

SKILLS:
A. Select the sensor and connect to patient, verify EtCO2 numerical value.
B. Verify continuous waveform
C. Continually monitor the patient and values and adjust interventions as needed.

SECTION 2 – LIFTING AND MOVING PATIENTS

OBJECTIVES:
- To provide mechanisms of patient movement and transport, which eliminate or minimize the potential for further patient injury while providing a rate of transport of movement appropriate to existing emergency conditions
- To provide mechanisms of patient movement and transport, which provide the greatest degree of patient and rescuer safety

1. EMERGENCY MOVES: When using emergency moves it is assumed the patient must be moved to a position of relative safety immediately and no time is available to begin an assessment or provide spinal immobilization

POINTS OF EMPHASIS:
- The greatest danger in moving a patient quickly is the potential of aggravating a spine injury
- Always pull in the direction of the long axis of the patient's body
- Do not pull a patient sideways; avoid bending or twisting the patient's torso
- The patient should be in a position to protect their airway and breathing

A. BLANKET DRAG
   1. Place patient on blanket
   2. Drag blanket in direction of long axis of patient's body
      a. Keep head as close to floor as possible
      b. Move patient head first whenever possible

B. CLOTHES DRAG
   1. Grasp patient's clothing pulling from the neck or shoulder area
   2. Drag in direction of the long axis of the patient's body
      a. Keep patient's head as close to the floor as possible
      b. Drag in direction of the long axis of the body

C. ONE-RESCUER DRAG
   1. Place hands under the patient's armpits from the back
   2. Grasp the patient's forearms and drag in the direction of the long axis of the body

URGENT MOVES: Urgent moves are required when the patient must be moved quickly but adequate time is available to perform an initial assessment and provide spinal immobilization precautions when necessary.

POINTS OF EMPHASIS:
- The greatest danger in moving a patient quickly is the potential of aggravating injuries
- Always pull in the direction of the long axis of the patient's body
- Do not pull a patient sideways; avoid bending or twisting the patient's torso.
- Manual C-spine stabilization may be done if time and personnel allow.
- Manual C-spine stabilization may need to be transferred between Diver Medics during patient transfer because of vehicular obstacles.
- To permit emergency extrication of a patient when their condition does not allow the time required to apply full head and torso immobilization with a short extrication device.

- To permit emergency extrication in a hazardous situation (fire, HazMat, etc.)
- To permit an alternative extrication technique when a short immobilization device is not available.

SKILLS:

A. RAPID EXTRICATION (Patient sitting in vehicle)

1. First rescuer brings cervical spine into neutral, in-line position and provides manual stabilization
2. Second rescuer applies cervical immobilization device (rigid cervical collar)
3. Third rescuer positions the foot-end of a long board at the door opening, then moves to opposite side of patient
4. Second rescuer supports and stabilizes the patient's torso as the third rescuer frees the patient's legs
5. At the direction of the rescuer holding manual C-spine stabilization, the patient is rotated in several short, coordinated moves until the patient's back is in the open doorway and his/her legs are on the seat
6. The foot end of the long board is placed against the patient's buttocks. Additional rescuers support the opposite end of the board as the first and second rescuers lower the patient to the board
7. The second and third rescuers slide the patient into the proper position on the board in short coordinated moves while the first rescuer maintains manual C-spine stabilization
8. First rescuer maintains manual stabilization as the patient is moved to a place of relative safety

B. BLANKET COLLAR EXTRICATION (Patient sitting)

SKILLS:
HORSE COLLAR EXTRICATION (patient sitting)

1. Hold a full size cloth blanket diagonally at opposite corners: Loosely swing like a jump rope to make a bulky, long cravat
2. Position the blanket for C-spine control and movement
    a. Place the middle of the blanket behind the patient's neck
    b. Bring the ends over the shoulders
    c. Cross the blanket in front of the chest
    d. Pass the ends under the armpits
    e. Cross the ends behind the patient's back
3. Hold the blanket ends close to the armpits
4. Tilt the patient's upper body to clear the doorframe as needed
5. Slide the patient off and lower into a sitting position onto the ground or directly on to a long board
6. Lower the patient to a supine position

III. NON-URGENT MOVES: Non-urgent moves are those moves, which are used when adequate time is available to perform a thorough assessment and provide all appropriate immobilization precautions

C. DIRECT GROUND LIFT (no suspected spinal injury)
1. Two or three rescuers line up on one side of the patient
2. Rescuers kneel on one knee (preferably the same knee for all rescuers)
3. The rescuer at the head places one arm under the patient's neck and shoulders while cradling the patient's head. S/he places the other hand under the patient's lower back

4. The second rescuer places one arm under the patient's knees and the other arm just above the patient's buttocks
5. If a third rescuer is available, s/he should place both arms under the patient's waist and the other rescuers should slide their arms either up to the mid-back or down to the buttocks as appropriate
6. On signal, the rescuers lift the patient to their knees and roll the patient toward their chests
7. On signal, the rescuers stand and move the patient to the stretcher
8. To lower the patient, the steps are reversed

D. EXTREMITY LIFT (no suspected spinal or extremity injuries – patient supine)
1. Properly position the stretcher beside the patient
2. One rescuer kneels at the patient's head and one kneels at the patient's side by the knees
3. The rescuer at the head places one hand under each of the patient's shoulders while the rescuer at the foot grasps the patients wrists and pulls the patient to a sitting position
4. The rescuer at the head slips his/her hands under the patient's arms and grasps the patient's wrists
5. The rescuer at the patient's feet places his/her hands under the patient's knees
6. Both rescuers move to a crouching position
7. Both rescuers stand simultaneously and move with the patient to the stretcher

E. SUPINE TRANSFER - Direct Carry
1. Position the stretcher perpendicular to the bed with the head end of the stretcher at the foot of the bed or the foot end of the stretcher at the head of the bed
2. Both rescuers stand between bed and stretcher, facing patient
3. First rescuer slides arm under patient's neck and cradles patient's head and shoulders
4. Second rescuer slides hands under patient's hips and lifts slightly
5. First rescuer slides other arm under patient's back
6. Second rescuer places arms under hips and calves
7. Rescuers slide patient to edge of bed
8. On signal, patient is lifted and curled toward rescuer's chests
9. Rescuers rotate and place patient gently on stretcher

F. SUPINE TRANSFER – Draw Sheet Method
1. Loosen bottom sheet beneath patient
2. Position stretcher next to and parallel to bed
3. Prepare stretcher and adjust to bed height
4. Rescuers then reach across stretcher and grasp sheet firmly at the patient's head, chest, hips and knees
5. On signal, slide the patient gently onto stretcher

G. STAND AND PIVOT (seated patient)

POINTS OF EMPHASIS:
1. The patient must be able to bear some weight
2. One or two rescuers may be used
3. Position the cot close to the patient with its height about the same as a chair seat
4. The patient may want to hold on to the shoulders of the Diver Medic's shoulders.
5. If the patient has footwear that will easily slide on the floors' surface, the Diver Medic may need to stand toe-to-toe with patient to prevent slipping.

SKILLS:
1. While facing the patient, grasp the patient by the waistband or under the armpits
2. On the rescuer's count, assist the patient to a standing position
3. Assist the patient in turning (pivoting) so their posterior is toward the cot
4. Once the patient's legs are touching the cot, lower the patient to a seated position
5. Position the patient on the cot

IV. EQUIPMENT MOVES:

1. Stair Chair- Follow manufacturer's instructions for proper use
2. Stretchers – Follow manufacturer's instructions for proper use
   a. Manual
   b. Powered
   c. Flexible
   d. Portable
3. Neonate Isolette
4. Child passenger safety seats
5. Vacuum mattress
6. Long and short backboards
7. Lifting devices for bariatric patients

SECTION 3 – AIRWAY AND RESPIRATORY MANAGEMENT

OBJECTIVES:
- To create a properly functioning oxygen delivery system, through the assembly of individual components, capable of providing appropriate oxygen concentrations for the purpose of patient resuscitation and inhalation therapy
- To provide the proper positioning of an unconscious patient for the purpose of maintaining patency of the patient's airway
- To facilitate the patency of a patient's airway through the use of basic and advanced airway adjuncts
- To create a properly functioning suction system, through the assembly of individual system components, capable of removing foreign materials, blood, fluids and bodily secretions from the upper airway
- To facilitate the removal of foreign body and/or displaced body tissues from the patient's upper airway through appropriate use of the Magill forceps and laryngoscope
- To provide adequate resuscitation and/or ventilatory assistance through the use of adjunct airway devices to include: the bag-valve-mask, pocket mask, and flow restricted oxygen powered ventilation device (FROPVD)

POINTS OF EMPHASIS:
- Always position the patient properly to assure an open airway
- Open the airway using the head-tilt/chin lift or jaw thrust maneuvers
- Modifications for maintaining the airway may be necessary due to the patient's injuries and/or condition
- Confirm a patent airway by observing chest rise and fall, and air exchange
- Artificial ventilation should never be delayed if airway adjuncts are not readily available or supplemental oxygen are not readily available.
- Auscultate lung sounds bilaterally to ensure adequacy.
- Be alert to changes in the patients' airway status.

I. OXYGEN ADMINISTRATION / DISCONTINUANCE

POINTS OF EMPHASIS:
- Oxygen cylinders must be handled carefully since the contents are under high pressure
- Selection of a delivery device will depend on the patient's condition
- Regulators reduce the cylinder's pressure to a safe level and regulate the flow of gas in liters per minute
- Cylinders should retain a safe residual volume of 500 psi or per local protocol.

SKILLS:
A. PREPARING OXYGEN TANK FOR USE
  1. Identify oxygen cylinder by color, correct pin code and 100% USP marking
  2. Remove protective cap or tape
  3. Quickly open and close cylinder valve to "crack" to remove any impurities, which may have accumulated on the mating surfaces between the tank and regulator
  4. Attach regulator and flowmeter and insure a leak-proof seal
  5. Turn on cylinder and check pressure gauge to insure adequate pressure
B. OXYGEN ADMINISTRATION

1. Attach appropriate delivery device to flowmeter
2. Adjust flow control to deliver recommended level
3. Fit delivery device to patient
4. Check adequacy of flow to patient

C. OXYGEN DISCONTINUANCE
1. Remove oxygen delivery device from patient
2. Shut off cylinder and bleed regulator
3. Return flowmeter control to "off" position

II. PATIENT POSITIONING (Non-trauma unresponsive patient)

POINTS OF EMPHASIS:
- This position may be useful for maintaining a patent airway and preventing aspiration in patients who are unable to properly protect their own airway
- Airway, ventilations and vital signs should be monitored continuously

SKILLS:
A. RECOVERY/LATERAL RECUMBANT POSITION
1. Roll the patient onto their side while supporting the head and neck
2. Flex uppermost leg and position knee to support weight
3. Position lower arm out behind patient or place lower arm and forearm under head for support
4. Position upper arm alongside patient's face to assist in supporting weight
5. Ease patient's head back and jut chin to facilitate airway

III. OROPHARYNGEAL AIRWAY INSERTION (Unresponsive patient with no gag reflex)

POINTS OF EMPHASIS:
- Always measure airway
- Use jaw thrust without head-tilt for patients with possible cervical spine injury
- Tongue depressor or similar device may be used to ease insertion
- Only to be used on a patient without a gag reflex.

SKILLS:
A. Select airway by measuring from the corner of the patient's lips to the bottom of the earlobe or angle of the jaw
B. Open mouth using cross-finger technique
C. Insert airway
   a. Adult only – with tip pointing toward roof of mouth, insert airway until point touches soft palette, rotate 180 degrees into position with flange resting against lips or teeth
   b. Adult, child or infant – Using a tongue depressor or similar device. Move the patient's tongue forward and down. Insert airway in anatomical position so as to follow the normal curvature of the oropharynx until the flange rests against the lips or teeth
D. Check for adequate air exchange

IV. NASOPHARYNGEAL AIRWAY INSERTION (Responsive or unresponsive patient)

POINTS OF EMPHASIS:
- If resistance is felt, remove and try other nare.
- Do not use in patients under one year of age.
- Do not use in patient with a suspected basilar skull fracture.

SKILLS:
  A. Visualize the nares and select a nasopharyngeal airway slightly smaller in diameter than the patient's largest nare
  B. Size the device by measuring from the tip of the patient's nose to the tip of the earlobe or angle of the jaw
  C. Lubricate the distal surface of the airway with water or a water soluble lubricant, being careful not to occlude the opening with lubricant.
  D. Insert the airway into the nare
      1. If placed in the right nare, insert following the normal anatomical curvature of the nasopharynx with the bevel toward the septum. Direct it along the floor of the nose and into the oropharynx
      2. If placed in the left nare, invert the airway so the bevel of the airway follows the septum of the nose. Once the tip of the airway reaches the nasopharynx, rotate the airway 180 degrees to resume alignment with the normal anatomical curvature of the nasopharynx. Continue to insert the airway into the oropharynx
  E. Check for adequate air exchange

V. NON-VISUALIZED ADVANCED AIRWAY INSERTION

POINTS OF EMPHASIS:
- EMR non-visualized airway insertion is allowed with specific training and approvals in accordance with DMO policy.
- Ventilate the patient per AHA guidelines for a minimum of thirty (30) seconds prior to attempting placement and between airway placement attempts.
- All indications and contraindications for airway use must be considered prior to insertion
- A maximum of thirty (30) seconds should be allowed for each airway attempt
- A maximum of three (3) attempts per patient to place airway may be made
- Confirm a patent airway by observing chest rise and fall, air exchange, and skin color.
- Artificial ventilation should never be delayed if airway adjuncts are not readily available.
- Placement of non-visualized airway is assessed through proper auscultation of epigastric and breath sounds.
    - Obtaining baseline breath sounds prior to advanced airway placement can assist with evaluation of airway placement
    - The presence of certain chest injuries (i.e. pneumothorax, hemothorax, etc.) will result in absent or diminished breath sounds on the affected side(s) even with proper airway placement.
    - Bilateral breath sounds and/or epigastric sounds, may or may not be present due to reasons other than incorrect airway placement.
- The ability to suction the airway must be constantly available when inserting or removing the airway. Suctioning of the airway should be done in accordance with the S & P.
- Gastric distention should be relieved by using gentle pressure on the abdomen or placement of a nasogastric tube.
- Place the patient in a neutral or sniffing position for insertion.
    - Use appropriate C-spine stabilization in cases of known or suspected c-spine trauma.

- Obese patients may need padding under shoulders and upper back.
- Use the tongue-jaw lift to open the airway.
  - The chin lift, laryngoscope, or tongue depressor can be used to lift the tongue anteriorly to allow easy advancement of the non-visualized airway.
- Always be certain that both syringes stay with the patient as long as s/he is intubated with a Combitube®.
- For the King LTS-D®:
  - It is important that the tip of the device be maintained at midline to assure that the distal tip is properly placed in the hypopharynx/upper esophagus.
  - During insertion, if the tip is placed or deflected laterally, it may enter the periform fossa and will appear to bounce back upon full insertion and release.
  - Insertion can be accomplished via a midline approach by applying a chin lift and sliding the distal tip along the palate and into position in the hypopharynx (head extension may be helpful)
- Local protocols may alter sequence in which epigastric and breath sounds are checked. Regardless of sequence, epigastric and bilateral breath sounds must be assessed for placement verification.
- When possible, have a partner ventilate the patient while preparing the equipment, during placement checks, and while securing the non-visualized airway.
- Be alert for changes in the patient's airway status.
- Placement should be reconfirmed frequently and after every patient move.
- Anticipate that the patient will vomit when removing the non-visualized airway.

SKILLS:

A. ESOPHAGEAL-TRACHEAL COMBITUBE® (ETC)

   1. INSERTION

      a. Reconfirm assessment of absent or inadequate breathing without a gag reflex.

      b. Determine cuff integrity

          1) Inflate cuffs

          2) Disconnect syringes

          3) Carefully inspect the pharyngeal and distal cuffs.

          4) Carefully inspect the valves and pilot cuffs.

          5) Deflate both cuffs

      c. Prepare all necessary accessories

          1) Preset inflation syringes to 100 ml and 15 ml (For Small Adult [SA] Model Preset to 85 ml and 12 ml)

          2) Bag-valve-mask with supplemental oxygen

          3) Water soluble lubricant

          4) Suction device

          5) Stethoscope

      d. Suction as necessary; inspect patient's airway for obstructions, broken teeth, dentures, dental appliances, tongue piercings, or other items that could damage the cuffs.

      e. Ventilate for a minimum of 30 seconds.

      f. Lubricate the tip of the Combitube®, avoiding any openings, with water-soluble lubricant as necessary.

      g. Position the patient supine with head in the neutral position. Do not hyperextend the patient's head .

      h. Remove the oropharyngeal airway if previously inserted.

      i. While holding the patient's tongue and lower jaw to facilitate insertion:

          1) Insert the Combitube® airway following the normal anatomical curvature of the oropharynx.

2) Insert firmly but gently until the insertion markers (two black lines which encircle the proximal end of the airway) are aligned on opposite sides of the patient's teeth or gums.
- (a) Do not use force – If airway does not insert easily, withdraw and reattempt
- (b) Ventilate for a minimum of thirty (30) seconds between attempts
- (c) Maximum of thirty (30) seconds for each attempt
- (d) Maximum of three (3) attempts
- (e) Suction as necessary between attempts

j. When Combitube® is positioned
1) Inflate the pharyngeal cuff with 100 mL of air using large syringe (85 mL for Small Adult [SA] Model) through line #1 (blue)
2) Insure Combitube® has remained in proper position. (Combitube® will move slightly with inflation)
3) Remove syringe and insure pharyngeal cuff inflation has occurred by observing pilot balloon
4) Inflate distal cuff with 15 mL of air using smaller syringe (12 mL for Small Adult [SA] Model) through line #2 (white)
5) Remove syringe and insure distal cuff inflation has occurred by observing pilot balloon

k. Ventilate the patient
1) Attach bag-valve-mask (BVM) to primary tube #1 (blue) and ventilate patient
2) While ventilating, confirm tube placement by auscultation of breath and epigastric sounds
- (a) Assess breath and epigastric sounds
  - i. Esophageal placement
    1) Breath sounds present high axillary
    2) Breath sounds present bilaterally
    3) Epigastric sounds are absent
    4) Continue to ventilate through tube #1 (blue)
  - ii. Tracheal placement
    - (1) Breath sounds are not present high axillary
    - (2) Breath sounds are not present bilaterally
    - (3) Epigastric sounds are present
    - (4) Discontinue ventilation through primary tube #1 (blue)
    - (5) Ventilate through secondary tube #2 (clear)
    - (6) Reassess breath and epigastric sounds to confirm tracheal placement
  - iii. Unknown placement
    - (1) Breath sounds are not present high axillary
    - (2) Breath sounds are not present bilaterally
    - (3) Epigastric sounds are not present
    - (4) Deflate cuffs (blue then white)
    - (5) Reposition airway – withdrawing approximately ½ inch
    - (6) Re-inflate cuffs with appropriate volume of air (blue then white)
    - (7) Begin ventilations through primary tube #1 (blue) and reassess breath and epigastric sounds to confirm placement
    - (8) Ventilate as appropriate
  - iv. Placement remains unknown
    - (1) Follow removal procedures
    - (2) Ventilate patient for minimum of thirty (30) seconds
    - (3) Reattempt placement (maximum of three (3) attempts) starting at the beginning of the insertion steps

2. REMOVAL
   a. Prepare suction and emesis collection devices
   b. Position patient in lateral recumbent position when feasible, observing appropriate C-spine precautions for trauma patients
   c. Use large syringe to deflate cuff #1 (blue) until pilot balloon is completely deflated
   d. Use small syringe to deflate cuff #2 (white) until pilot balloon is completely deflated
   e. Immediately withdraw airway with a smooth and steady motion while maintaining normal curvature of the pharynx
   f. Suction as necessary
   g. Monitor the patient's airway and breathing closely
   h. Provide high-flow oxygen via non-rebreather mask
   i. Consider nasopharyngeal airway and assist ventilations as necessary

B. KING LTS-D ADVANCED AIRWAY
   1. INSERTION
      a. Reconfirm assessment of absent or inadequate breathing without a gag reflex
      b. Determine correct size airway based on patient's height
      c. Determine cuff integrity
         i. Inflate cuffs
         ii. Disconnect syringes
         iii. Carefully inspect pharyngeal and distal cuff
         iv. Carefully inspect valve and pilot cuff
         v. Deflate cuffs
      d. Prepare all necessary accessories
         i. Preset inflation syringe to correct amount for device size
         ii. Bag-valve-mask with supplemental oxygen
         iii. Water soluble lubricant
         iv. Suction device
         v. Stethoscope
      e. Suction as necessary; inspect patient's airway for obstructions, broken teeth, dentures, dental appliances, tongue piercings or other items that could damage cuffs
      f. Ventilate for a minimum of thirty (30) seconds
      g. Lubricate airway with water soluble lubricant as necessary
      h. Position the patient supine with head in the neutral or sniffing position. Do not hyperextend the patient's head

   2. NORMAL INSERTION
      a. Hold the King LTS-D at the connector with dominant hand
      b. With non-dominant hand, hold mouth open and apply chin lift unless contraindicated by C-spine precautions or patient position
      c. Using a lateral approach, introduce the tip into the corner of the mouth
      d. Advance the tip behind the base of the tongue while rotating the tube back to midline so that the blue orientation line faces the chin of the patient
      e. Without exerting excessive force, advance tube until base of connector is aligned with teeth or gums
      f. Deeper placement and subsequent retraction is preferred
      g. When the King LTS-D is positioned
         i. Inflate cuffs to volume sufficient to seal the airway
         ii. Attach ventilation device to the connector of the King LTS-D

iii. At the same time, gently bag the patient and withdraw the King LTS-D until ventilation is easy and free flowing
   iv. Readjust cuff inflation to "just seal" volume
   v. Check breath sounds, epigastric sounds and chest rise and fall
3. SECURE THE AIRWAY
   a. Disconnect the ventilation device
   b. Aggressively tape the King LTS-D in the midline to the maxilla
   c. Avoid taping over gastric access lumen
   d. Reattach the ventilation device
4. REMOVAL
   a. Remove the King LTS-D when protective reflexes have returned
   b. Prepare suction and emesis collection devices – suction as indicated
   c. Position patient in lateral recumbent position when feasible, observing appropriate C-spine precautions for trauma patients
   d. Deflate cuffs
   e. Immediately withdraw airway with a smooth and steady motion while maintaining normal curvature of the pharynx
   f. Monitor the patient's airway and breathing closely
   g. Provide high-flow oxygen via non-rebreather mask
   h. Consider nasopharyngeal airway and assist ventilations as necessary

VI. ENDOTRACHEAL TUBE INSERTION AND REMOVAL

POINTS OF EMPHASIS
- Ventilate the patient per AHA guidelines for a minimum of 30 seconds prior to attempting placement and between airway placement attempts.
- All indications and contraindications for airway use must be considered prior to insertion.
- A maximum of thirty (30) seconds should be allowed for each airway attempt.
- A maximum of three (3) airway attempts per patient to place airway may be made.
- Confirm patent airway with chest rise and fall, and air exchange, and skin color.
- Artificial ventilation should never be delayed if airway adjuncts are not readily available.
- Follow department guidelines for which medications may be used to facilitate intubation.
- Two paramedics must be at patient side when administering paralytics.
- Position the patient properly to assure an open airway.
   a. Placement of padding under the occiput may help with proper alignment.
   b. Placement of padding under the shoulders of a small child or infant may help with proper alignment.
- Placement of endotracheal tube (ET) is assessed through primary and secondary methods.
   a. Obtaining baseline breath sounds and epigastric sounds prior to advanced airway placement can assist with evaluation of tube placement.
   b. The presence of certain chest injuries (pneumothorax, hemothorax, etc.) will result in absent or diminished breath sounds on the affected side(s) even with proper placement.
   c. Bilateral breath sounds and/or epigastric sounds, may or may not be present due to reasons of incorrect tube placement.
   d. Use a secondary device (EtCO2, colorimetric device) to confirm and monitor placement of the ET.
   e. Correlate secondary placement device with the patient's condition and assessment findings. Rule out possibility of false positive and false negative findings.

- The ability to suction the airway must be constantly available when inserting or removing the airway. Suctioning of the oropharynx should be done in accordance with this S&P Manual.
- Local protocols may alter the sequence in which epigastric and breath sounds are checked. Regardless of the sequence, epigastric and bilateral breath sounds must be assessed for placement verification.
- Be alert for changes in the patient's airway status.
- Placement should be reconfirmed frequently and after every patient move.
- Rescue airway should be readily in case intubation is unsuccessful.
- When possible, have a partner ventilate the patient while preparing equipment, during placement checks, and securing the ET.
- For nasotracheal placement:
    a. Do not use in patients with suspected basal skull fracture.
    b. The patient must be breathing.
    c. Typically the nasotracheal tube size is one size smaller than the orotracheal tube size.
- Anticipate secretions from vomiting and/or coughing when removing an ET tube.

SKILLS

A. OROTRACHEAL INTUBATION INSERTION
1. Reconfirm assessment foe need of endotracheal intubation.
2. Prepare all necessary equipment and accessories.
    a. Cuff (determine cuff integrity then deflate.)
    b. Syringe (preset inflation syringe according to manufacturer instructions)
    c. Laryngoscope and blade (check for functioning light)
    d. Stylet (stylet tip must be recessed from the tip of the tube)
    e. Bag-valve-mask with supplemental oxygen
    f. Water soluble lubricant to lubricate tip as needed.
    g. Suction device
    h. Stethoscope
    i. Securing device
    j. Secondary device for endotracheal confirmation.
    k. Other accessories that will be used such as Bougie, video scope, medications.
3. Suction as necessary; inspect patient's airway for obstructions, broken teeth, dentures, dental appliances, tongue piercings, or other items that could damage the cuff.
4. Ventilate for a minimum of thirty (30) seconds
5. Position the patient's head properly. Do not hyperextend the patient's head.
    a. For patients without suspected spinal injury, place in sniffing position with the head tilted and neck extended.
    b. For patients with possible spinal injuries, maintain inline cervical spine stabilization during the entire intubation process.
6. Remove the oropharyngeal airway if previously inserted
7. When positioned superior to the patient's head, insert laryngoscope blade into the right side of the patient's mouth while displacing the tongue to the left.
8. Elevate the mandible with laryngoscope to visualize the vocal cords
    a. Insert endotracheal tube, following the normal anatomical curvature of the oropharynx
    b. Insert firmly but gently until the cuff is distal to the vocal cords
        1) Do not force – if airway does not easily, withdraw and reattempt
        2) Ventilate for a minimum of thirty (30) seconds between attempts
        3) Maximum of thirty (30) seconds per attempt

            4) Maximum of three (3) attempts
            5) Suction as necessary between attempts
    9. When endotracheal tube is positioned.
        a. Inflate the cuff with minimal amount of air to prevent air leaks.
        b. Ensure the ET tube has remained in the proper position.
        c. Remove syringe and ensure cuff inflation has occurred by observing the pilot balloon.
    10. Maintain manual stabilization of ET tube until secured.
    11. Ventilate the patient confirming proper placement
        a. Ideally attach capnography or a CO2 colorimetric device before the first ventilation.
        b. Attach a bag-valve-mask (BVM) to ET tube and ventilate the patient
        c. While ventilating, listen over the stomach.
    12. Confirm proper placement through primary and secondary methods
        a. Tracheal placement
            1) No epigastric sounds auscultated during ventilations
            2) Breath sounds present bilaterally
            3) Secure endotracheal tube
        b. Esophageal placement
            1) If you hear epigastric sounds, stop ventilating, remove tube, and continue to manage the airway
        c. Right main stem placement
            1) Epigastric sounds are NOT present
            2) Breath sounds are present on the right
            3) Breath sounds are NOT present on the left
            4) Deflate cuff
            5) Withdraw endotracheal tube 1-2 cm
            6) Re-inflate cuff with appropriate volume of air
            7) Begin ventilations and reassess epigastric and breath sounds to confirm placement
            8) Ventilate as appropriate
        d. Unknown placement
            1) Epigastric sounds are not present
            2) Breath sounds are not present high axillary
            3) Breath sounds are not present bilaterally
                a) Deflate the cuff
                b) Reposition endotracheal tube
                c) Begin ventilations and reassess epigastric and breath sounds to confirm placement
                d) Ventilate as appropriate
            4) Placement remains unknown
                a) Remove endotracheal tube
                b) Ventilate patient for a minimum of thirty (30) seconds
                c) Reattempt placement (maximum three (3) attempts
    13. When placement is confirmed, secure endotracheal tube with tape or commercial device

B. NASOTRACHEAL INTUBATION INSERTION
    1. Reconfirm assessment for need of endotracheal intubation
    2. Assess the nares and select the larger for intubation
    3. Prepare the necessary equipment and accessories
        a. Cuff (determine cuff integrity and then deflate)
        b. Syringe (preset inflation syringe to manufacturer's instructions)

      c. Bag-valve-mask with supplemental oxygen
      d. Water soluble lubricant to lubricate tip as needed.
      e. Suction device
      f. Stethoscope
      g. Securing device or tape
      h. Secondary device for endotracheal confirmation
4. Suction as necessary; inspect patient's airway for obstruction
5. Ventilate for minimum thirty (30) seconds
6. Maintain patient's head in a neutral position
7. Remove oropharyngeal or nasopharyngeal airway if previously inserted
8. Insert ET tube into selected nare with the bevel towards the septum until reaching the bridge of the nose. If using the right nare, continue with insertion; if using the left nare, rotate the ET tube to follow the normal curvature of the airway
      a. Advance the ET tube straight back along the floor of the nasal passage until the tip is just above the vocal cords. Air movement can be heard through the tube.
      b. When the patient inhales, insert the ET tube firmly but gently; advance until the flange of the ET tube rest against the nare.
      c. If resistance is met, remove, and attempt placement in the other nare
            1) Do not use force – If the airway does not insert easily, withdraw and reattempt
            2) Ventilate for a minimum of thirty (30) seconds between attempts
            3) Maximum thirty (30) seconds per attempt
            4) Maximum three (3) attempts
            5) Suction as needed between attempts
9. When endotracheal tube is positioned
      a. Inflate the cuff with minimal air to prevent air leaks
      b. Ensure the ET tube remains in position
      c. Remove the syringe and ensure the cuff inflation has occurred by observing the pilot balloon
10. Maintain manual stabilization of the ET tube until secured
11. Ventilate the patient confirming proper placement
      a. Ideally attach capnography or a CO_2 colorimetric device before the first ventilation
      b. Attach a bag-valve-mask (BVM) to ET tube and ventilate the patient
      c. While ventilating, auscultate over the epigastrium
12. Confirm proper placement through primary and secondary methods
      a. Tracheal placement
            1) No epigastric sounds auscultated with ventilations
            2) Breath sounds present bilaterally
            3) Secure endotracheal tube
      b. Esophageal placement
            1) If you hear epigastric sounds, stop ventilating, remove the tube, and continue to manage the airway
      c. Right main stem placement
            1) Epigastric sounds not present
            2) Breath sounds present on the right
            3) Breath sounds not present on the left
            4) Deflate cuff
            5) Withdraw tube approximately 1-2 cm
            6) Re-inflate cuff with appropriate volume of air
            7) Begin ventilations and reassess epigastric and breath sounds to confirm placement
            8) Ventilate as appropriate

    d. Unknown placement
        1) Epigastric sounds not present
        2) Breath sounds are not present high axillary
        3) Breath sounds are not present bilaterally
            a) Deflate cuff
            b) Reposition endotracheal tube
            c) Re-inflate cuff with appropriate volume of air
            d) Begin ventilations and reassess epigastric and breath sounds to confirm placement
            e) Ventilate as appropriate
    e. Placement remains unknown
        1) Remove endotracheal tube
        2) Ventilate the patient for a minimum of thirty (30) seconds
        3) Reattempt placement (maximum three (3) attempts)
13. When placement is confirmed, secure endotracheal tube with tape or commercial device

C. ENDOTRACHEAL TUBE REMOVAL / EXTUBATION
1. Recognize need for extubation
2. Prepare suction and emesis collection devices
3. Position patient in upright or semi-Fowler's position
4. Explain procedure to patient
5. Oxygenate patient for one (1) minute, if possible
6. Suction secretions from oropharynx and mouth
7. Attach syringe to pilot balloon and deflate cuff while patient takes a deep breath
8. Instruct the patient to cough as the tube is pulled gently, but quickly
9. Provide supplemental oxygen and encourage the patient to take deep breaths
10. Monitor respiratory status carefully

VII. PHARYNGEAL AND TRACHEOBRONCHIAL SUCTIONING

POINTS OF EMPHASIS
- Always measure flexible catheters
- Use cross-finger technique or tongue blade devices to prevent Diver Medic and/or patient injury
- Apply suction after reaching the insertion depth
- Maximum suction time for adults is 15 seconds
- Maximum suction time for pediatric patients is 5 seconds
- Suction the mouth first, then the nose on infants
- Determining the depth of insertion for suction catheters
    - Rigid tip: Do not lose sight of the distal tip
    - Flexible tip: Measure from tip of the earlobe to the corner of the mouth
    - Tracheobronchial suction: There are many acceptable ways to perform this skill, follow company and/or DMO approved policies
- Suction unit should be set to 80-120 mmHg when using an open- suction system. If using a closed suction system, follow the manufacturer's direction.

SKILLS
A. FLEXABLE/RIGID TIP
    1. Attach suction tip to suction device

2. Switch on suction unit (or begin pumping) and ensure suction is present
3. Open mouth using cross-finger technique or tongue blade
4. Insert suction tip to the proper depth into oropharynx with no suction at the tip
5. Initiate suction and suction across oropharynx
6. Remove suction tip while maintaining suction
7. Flush the system as needed
8. Check for adequate air exchange

B. BULB SYRINGE
1. Squeeze air from bulb prior to insertion
2. Gradually reduce pressure on the bulb to provide suction while removing from nose or mouth
3. Check for adequate air exchange
4. Repeat as necessary

C. TRACHEOBRONCHIAL SUCTIONING (endotracheal tube)
1. Pre-oxygenate patient for 30-60 seconds prior to each pass of the suction catheter when feasible
2. Attach flexible suction tip to suction device
3. Switch on suction unit and ensure suction is present
4. Measure or identify insertion length of the catheter by rough approximation or measuring against another endotracheal tube to determine insertion length. Use thumb and one finger to mark the insertion length
5. Use the other hand to feed catheter into endotracheal tube without suction
6. Once catheter is at desired insertion depth, create suction and withdraw suction catheter with a rotating / twisting technique from the endotracheal tube (maximum 15 seconds for adult patient)
7. Remove device while maintaining suction
8. Flush system with sterile water or sterile saline until tubing is clear
9. Once lower airway is adequately cleared of secretions, perform oropharyngeal suctioning
10. Check for adequate air exchange

VIII. LARYNGOSCOPE AND MAGILL FORCEPS

POINTS OF EMPHASIS
- The laryngoscope is never levered against the teeth
- The Magill forceps should be held in the right hand so the handle does not obstruct the view of the pharynx
- Curved blades are to be used for foreign body removal
- This device is intended to be used on unconscious patients

SKILLS
A. Choose appropriate-sized forceps, laryngoscope handle and blade per manufacturer's specification
B. Assemble blade and handle, ensure the light is bright and tightly secured in the blade
C. Place the patient's head in the 'sniffing' position
D. Hold the laryngoscope in the left hand
    1. Adult patient – Hold handle with the entire hand
    2. Infant patient – Hold handle with thumb, index and middle fingers while supporting the chin with ring and little fingers of left hand for leverage
E. With the Diver Medic at the patient's head, insert the blade into the right side of the mouth and displace the tongue to the left by moving to the midline
F. Lift tongue in direction of the long axis of the handle without prying on the teeth or gums
G. Visualize the obstruction

H. Using the Magill forceps in the right hand, remove the obstruction
I. Visualize airway for further obstructions before removing the laryngoscope blade
J. Check for adequate air exchange

IX. BAG-VALVE-MASK (BVM)

POINTS OF EMPHASIS
- This device should be used with supplemental oxygen to delivery high concentrations of oxygen
- Inflate only enough to see visible chest rise
- The bag-valve-mask maybe used on patients who are not breathing or patients who are breathing but not exchanging adequate amounts of air
- Do not delay breathing to attach supplemental oxygen
- This procedure should be performed using the two Diver Medic technique whenever possible
- Appropriate C-spine considerations should be taken when managing patients with potential spinal injuries
- Pediatric bag-valve-mask devices may have a pop-off valve

SKILLS
A. Select and insert the appropriate airway adjunct
B. Select adult, pediatric, or infant sized bag-valve-mask and assemble components
C. Attach oxygen supply to bag-valve-mask
D. Seal the mask on the patient's face while maintaining head-tilt, chin-lift or attach to advanced airway adjunct fitting
E. Squeeze bag, ventilating patient per AHA guidelines
F. Observe chest rise and fall with each ventilation. If no chest rise, reassess equipment, technique and patient
G. If two Diver Medics are available, one DMT uses two hands to maintain the airway and mask seal, while the second DMT uses two hands to compress the bag to provide ventilations

X. MANUALLY TRIGGERED VENTILATION DEVICES

POINTS OF EMPHASIS
- Prolonged depression of the ventilation button may lead to gastric distention
- Proper airway positioning minimizes the potential for gastric distention
- Manually triggered ventilation devices are not recommended for use on pediatric patients or chest trauma patients
- Must be reduced or restricted to deliver no more than 40 LPM of oxygen
- May be used by spontaneously breathing patients
- Follow company and/or DMO protocols governing the use of this device
- Appropriate C-spine considerations should be taken when managing patients with potential spine injuries

SKILLS
A. Connect device to oxygen source
B. Open cylinder and check for leaks
C. Select and insert appropriate airway adjunct, if indicated

D. Press ventilation button to clear line and check operation
E. Seal mask on patient's face while maintaining head-tilt, chin-lift or attach to advanced airway adjunct fitting
F. Depress ventilation button until patient's chest rises
G. Release ventilation button and observe patient's exhalation
H. Ventilate per AHA guidelines

XI. POCKET MASK

POINTS OF EMPHASIS
- Oxygen concentrations will be increased by attaching supplemental oxygen
- Do not delay ventilations to connect supplemental oxygen
- Remove one-way valve when attaching bag-valve-mask device
- Appropriate C-spine considerations should be taken when managing patients with potential spine injuries

SKILLS
A. Select and insert the appropriately sized oropharyngeal airway or nasopharyngeal airway, if available
B. Unfold pocket mask as appropriate and attach one-way valve
C. If available, attach oxygen tubing and supply to oxygen inlet on mask
D. Turn on oxygen and adjust liter flow to recommended level
E. While maintaining head-tilt, chin-lift, seal mask to patient's face
F. Ventilate patient through the one-way valve attached to the mask until the chest rises
G. Allow the patient to exhale while maintaining the mask seal
H. Ventilate per AHA guidelines

XII. CONTINUOUS POSITIVE AIR PRESSURE

POINT OF EMPHASIS
- All indications and contraindications for use of CPAP must be considered

SKILLS
A. APPLICATION
    1. Explain the procedure to the patient
    2. Ensure adequate oxygen supply to ventilate device
    3. Place patient on continuous pulse oximetry
    4. Place the patient on a cardiac monitor (if available) and record rhythm strips along with vital signs
    5. Place the delivery device over the mouth and nose
    6. Secure the mask with the provide straps or other provided devices
    7. Use appropriate cm H2O of PEEP per protocol
    8. Check for air leaks
    9. Monitor and document the patient's respiratory response to treatment
    10. Check and document vital signs every 5 minutes
    11. Administer appropriate medication as certified (continuous nebulized albuterol for COPD/asthma and repeated administration of nitroglycerin spray or tablets for CHF)
    12. Continue to coach the patient to keep the mask in-place and readjust as needed
    13. Request ALS assistance if available

14. If respiratory status deteriorates, remove the device and consider intermittent positive pressure ventilation using a BVM and/or placement of a non-visualized airway or endotracheal tube.

B. REMOVAL PROCEDURE

1. CPAP therapy needs to be continuous and should not be removed unless the patient cannot tolerate the mask or experiences respiratory arrest or begins to vomit
2. Intermittent positive pressure ventilation with a BVM, placement of a non-visualized airway and/or endotracheal intubation should be considered if the patient is removed from CPAP therapy

XIII. PERCUTANEOUS SURGICAL / NEEDLE CRICOTHYROTOMY

OBJECTIVE:
- To provide an emergent airway via a surgical or needle cricothyrotomy when unable to manage the airway by any other means

POINT OF EMPHASIS
- Complete patient assessment must be performed to determine the patient needs an emergent cricothyrotomy
- To minimize risk of infection, prep the area of puncture and maintain sterility of equipment
- Administer 100% oxygen, and/or BVM ventilate the patient
- Gather equipment before starting the procedure and maintain sterility of equipment. Equipment may be a kit and/or include:
    - 14 gauge or larger needle for adult; 18 or 20 gauge for pediatric patient
    - Antimicrobial cleaning solution for cleansing site
    - 3.0 mm and 7.0 mm endotracheal tube adapters
    - Syringes ranging from 3 ml and 10 ml
    - Scalpel
    - Hemostats, small rake retractors or tracheal hook
    - Twill-tape or umbilical tape
    - Jet insufflator and/or BVM
    - 7.0 mm endotracheal tube or a tracheostomy tube for an adult; 5.0 mm for a pediatric patient
    - Stethoscope
    - EtCO2 detector
    - Sharps container
- Surgical cricothyrotomy
    - Not recommended for patients under 12 years of age
    - A vertical midline incision may result in a small amount of venous bleeding but avoids the lateral vasculature of the neck
    - A distinct "pop" will be felt as the scalpel pierces the membrane and enters the trachea
    - If the incision is lost, the location can be identified by means of air bubbles produced during exhalation. If the patient is apneic, apply pressure to the anterior chest wall to simulate exhalation and thereby producing the bubbles
- Document procedure and results, including any unusual circumstances and/or difficulties encountered.

SKILLS:
A. NEEDLE CRICOTHYROTOMY
   1. Place patient in a supine position
   2. Identify anatomical landmarks
      a. Palpate the thyroid cartilage (the first prominent landmark on the anterior neck) the cricoid cartilage (caudal to the thyroid cartilage), and the area between them, which is the cricothyroid space that contains the membrane
      b. With the non-dominant hand, stabilize the area using the first and third digits on either side of the thyroid cartilage, leaving the index finger to palpate the membrane
   3. Prep the area with antimicrobial solution
   4. Don sterile gloves
   5. Attach a 14 gauge or larger over-the-needle catheter to a 5 to 10 ml syringe
   6. Use the non-dominant hand, with sterile glove on, to re-identify anatomic landmarks and stabilize the puncture area
   7. Puncture the skin midline and directly over the cricothyroid membrane while stabilizing the trachea
   8. Direct the needle at a 45 degree angle caudally
   9. Carefully advance the needle through the cricothyroid membrane with constant aspiration (aspiration of air indicates entry into the tracheal lumen)
   10. Withdraw the metal needle while gently advancing the plastic catheter
   11. While using oxygen
      a. If using jet insufflator: connect catheter to jet insufflator (50 psi or 15 L/min) with the inspiratory/expiratory ratio set at 1:2
      b. If using a BVM device: attach the catheter to either a 3mm ET tube adapter or combine the barrel of a 3 mm syringe and a 7 mm ET tube adapter and ventilate using a BVM device
   12. Confirm placement through primary and secondary methods
   13 Secure the apparatus to the patient's neck
   14. Dispose of contaminated equipment in appropriate receptacle
   15. Continuously monitor and reassess patient for desired and undesired effects

B. SURGICAL CRICOTHYROTOMY
   1. Place the patient in a supine position
   2. Identify the anatomic landmarks
      a. Palpate the thyroid cartilage (the first prominent landmark on the anterior neck) the cricoid cartilage (caudal to the thyroid cartilage), and the area between them, which is the cricothyroid space that contains the membrane
      b. With the non-dominant hand, stabilize the area using the first and third digits on either side of the thyroid cartilage, leaving the index finger to palpate the membrane
   3. Prep the area with antimicrobial solution
   4. Don sterile gloves
   5. With the dominant hand, make a vertical incision midline, approximately 3 cm long and skin deep, over the cricothyroid membrane
   6. Palpate the cricothyroid membrane through the incision, using the index finger of the non-dominant hand
   7. Make a horizontal stab incision through the membrane
   8. Insert a tracheal hook or rake retractor at the superior end of the incision and retract the skin and membrane cephalically. Keep the scalpel in place until the tracheal hook or rake is inserted
   9. Insert the appropriately sized endotracheal tube or tracheostomy tube directing it caudally
   10. Inflate the cuff and ventilate the patient with a BVM device

11. Confirm placement by chest rise, auscultation over epigastrium, and bilaterally over the lungs while using waveform EtCO2 if available, to monitor the patient's real time cellular perfusion
12. Dispose of contaminated equipment in appropriate receptacle
13. Continually reassess patient for desired / undesired effect

SECTION 4 – PATIENT ASSESSMENT

The assessment process recognizes that trauma patients and medical patients have different assessment priorities. Patients may be divided into four broad categories: Medical patients who are responsive; Medical patients who are not responsive; Trauma patients with a significant mechanism of injury (MOI); and, Trauma patients without a significant mechanism of injury. Trauma patients are assigned a category based on severity, or potential severity, of their injuries. Medical patients, on the other hand, are assigned based on their ability to participate, or not participate, in the assessment rather than on the severity of their illnesses.

OBJECTIVES:
- To determine the presence or absence of actual or potential hazards which pose a threat to the health and safety of rescuers, patients or bystanders during rescuer operations and/or during transport
- To determine the presence or absence of injury or illness through a systematic assessment process incorporating inspection, auscultation, palpation, and the taking of a patient history

POINTS OF EMPHASIS
- Safety is paramount throughout the call
- Scene size-up and primary assessment must be completed prior to the secondary assessment
- MOI / NOI determines the path of assessment
- Patients with altered mental status include those who are unresponsive and those unable to respond reliably or provide history
- Intervene immediately to correct any life-threatening problem
- If the patient becomes unstable at any time, immediately repeat the initial assessment

SKILL:

I. PATIENT ASSESSMENT

A. SCENE SIZE-UP

1. Determine the Nature of Illness (NOI) or Mechanism of Injury (MOI)
    a. En route to scene:
        - Dispatch information
        - Other units at scene
    b. Upon arrival at scene:
        - Inspect the scene
        - Patient, family, witnesses, bystanders, other rescuers
2. Use appropriate body substance isolation precautions
3. Determine whether the scene is safe
    a. Environmental considerations
    b. Social considerations
    c. Crime scene considerations
    d. Unruly or violent persons
    e. Unstable surfaces
    f. Other hazards
    g. If the scene is not safe, make it safe, or do not enter

4. Determine the number of patients
5. Determine the need for, and request, additional resources prior to patient contact
6. Recognize the need for C-spine precautions

B. INITIAL ASSESSMENT

1. Form a general impression of the patient as you approach, while telling the patient your first name and explaining that you are an MEDIC
    a. Establish approximate age
    b. Establish gender
    c. Identify race
    d. Assess environment clues
    e. Identify any obvious life-threatening conditions requiring urgent intervention
2. Assess the patient's mental status and provide C-spine stabilization as appropriate
    a. Speak to the patient
        1) AVPU
            a) Alert
            b) Verbal
            c) Pain
            d) Unresponsive
3. Assess the patient's airway
    a. Is the patient talking or crying?
        1) Yes: Assess breathing
        2) No: Open airway
4. Assess the patient's breathing
    a. If the patient is not responsive, but breathing is adequate, open and maintain the airway and initiate oxygen therapy
    b. If the patient is not breathing adequately, open and maintain the airway, initiate oxygen therapy, utilize appropriate adjuncts and/or assist ventilations
    c. If the patient is not breathing, open and maintain the airway, utilize appropriate adjuncts and ventilate with supplemental oxygen
5. Assess the patient's circulation
    a. Pulse - present
        1) Less than one-year-old: Palpate the brachial artery
        2) More than one-year-old and responsive: Palpate the radial artery
        3) More than one-year-old and unresponsive; or more than one-year-old with absent radial pulse: Palpate carotid pulse
    b. If pulse - absent
        1) Initiate CPR
        2) Implement AED protocol as appropriate
    c. Assess and control major external bleeding
    d. Assess skin color, temperature and condition (Assess capillary refill in patients under six years or age)
6. Establish a field impression and differential diagnosis
7. Expose the patient, as needed and integrate life-saving interventions as needed
8. Evaluate patient stability and priority of patient care
9. Determine the patient's transport priority, consider ALS back-up

NOTE: The sequence in which History-Taking and Vital Signs are performed or when Monitoring Devices are used may depend on the circumstances, the number of available EMS providers and the presence of life-threatening problems requiring urgent intervention. Remember: The patient's priority is constantly being evaluated and subject to change.

C. Begin History-Taking
　　1. Investigate the chief complaint utilizing various sources such as the patient, family, bystanders, medical identification jewelry
　　2. Obtain statistical and demographic information such as correct dates, age, gender, race
　　3. Obtain current health status relative to tobacco and alcohol use, diet, immunizations
　　4. Obtain history of past/present illness (SAMPLE)
　　　　a. Signs and symptoms
　　　　b. Allergies
　　　　　　1) Medicines
　　　　　　2) Foods
　　　　　　3) Environmental
　　　　c. Medications
　　　　　　1) Prescriptions
　　　　　　2) Over-the-counter
　　　　　　3) Alternative medication, herbal supplements
　　　　d. Pertinent/past medical history
　　　　　　1) Heart disease
　　　　　　2) Diabetes
　　　　　　3) Seizures
　　　　　　4) Recent hospitalizations
　　　　　　5) Recent injuries
　　　　　　6) Medical patients: previous similar episodes
　　　　e. Last oral intake
　　　　f. Events leading to the injury or illness

　　5. Assess history of present injury or illness (OPQRST)
　　　　a. Onset
　　　　b. Provocation
　　　　c. Quality
　　　　d. Radiation
　　　　e. Severity
　　　　f. Timing
　　6. Additional questions pertinent to the present illness

D. Assess baseline vital signs
　　1. Breathing rate, rhythm, and quality
　　2. Pulse rate, rhythm, and quality
　　3. Blood pressure
　　4. Pupils
　　5. Skin color and temperature and condition

E. Use monitoring devices as needed
　　1. Pulse oximeter
　　2. Blood glucose monitor
　　3. Automated blood pressure measuring device
　　4. Other devices

F. Secondary Assessment
- 1. Perform an appropriate physical examination
    - a. Rapid physical (full body) scan (If not done in primary assessment)
        - 1) Used for unresponsive medical or trauma patient with significant MOI
        - 2) Assess for DCAP/BTLS
            - a) Deformities or dislocation
            - b) Contusions
            - c) Abrasions
            - d) Punctures / penetrations
            - e) Burns
            - f) Tenderness
            - g) Lacerations
            - h) Swelling
    - b. Focused assessment
        - 1) Used for responsive medical or trauma patient with no significant MOI
        - 2) Based on the patient's chief complaint
        - 3) Narrows exam to injury location or medical complaint
    - c. Secondary Assessment
        - 1) Head-to-Toe, slower, more deliberate assessment
        - 2) May be performed at scene, during transport or may be prohibitive depending upon patient care and condition
- 2. Establish a management plan and continue / initiate appropriate interventions
- 3. Revaluate transport decision

G. Reassessment
- 1. Repeat primary assessment
- 2. Reassess and record vital signs every 5 minutes (unstable patient) every 15 minutes (stable patient)
- 3. Repeat physical assessment as appropriate for patient
- 4. Reassess interventions and patient's response to treatment, revise as needed

SECTION 5 – CARDIAC MANAGEMENT

I. CARDIOPULMONARY RESUSCITATION

All cardiopulmonary resuscitation (CPR) procedures shall be performed as directed in the current American Heart Association (AHA) guidelines

II. AUTOMATED EXTERNAL DEFIBRILLATION

All AED procedures shall be performed as directed by the current AHA guidelines in concurrence with local protocols and/or medical direction

III. ELECTRICAL THERAPY

All electrical therapy shall be performed as directed by the current AHA guidelines in concurrence with local protocols and/or medical direction

OBJECTIVES:
- To safely provide electrical therapy for life-threatening emergencies.
- To deliver electrical energy through defibrillation.
- To deliver electrical energy through synchronized cardioversion.
- To deliver electrical energy through transcutaneous pacing.

GENERAL PRINCIPLES

- Always ensure good adhesion of defibrillator pads to the patient.
- An IV/IO should be started (if within the scope of practice) when electrical energy is needed.
- The appropriate sized defibrillation pads/paddles should be used. However, if pediatric pads/paddles are not available, adult pads/paddles should be used on a pediatric patient.
- Electrical energy should be used in conjunction with medications according to AHA guidelines (if within scope of practice).
- Hands free defibrillation is safest.
- When placing pre-gelled pads, roll the pads onto the prepped area. Press firmly on the adhesive and gently on the gelled area to remove trapped air and ensure good skin contact.
- Do not place defibrillation pads/paddles and pacing pads over an implanted pacer or cardioverter-defibrillation generator, medication patches, ECG cables and electrodes or dressings.

A. MANUAL DEFIBRILLATION

POINTS OF EMPHASIS
- Assess the environment for safety concerns when performing defibrillation (patient clear of fluids/puddles, good adherence of defibrillation pads, etc.
- Complete patient assessment to determine that patient is in cardiac arrest.
- Prep the area where the pads are to be applied by drying the skin, removing debris, minimizing hair, etc.

- Select defibrillation energy per AHA guidelines and manufacturer recommendations for the model defibrillator.
- Always verbally and visually clear the patient prior to defibrillating the patient.
- Assure high quality CPR is performed according to AHA guidelines.
- Initiate an IV/IO as soon as possible; do not delay defibrillation to initiate vascular access.
- Manual paddles
  - Paddles may allow operator to change energy level and may offer a "quick look" feature.
  - Defibrillation through paddles is achieved by simultaneously depressing both defibrillation buttons on the paddles.

SKILLS:
1. Confirm the absence of patient pulses
2. Direct partner(s) to initiate high quality CPR
3. Turn on monitor/defibrillator and check that defibrillation cable is attached to the unit.
4. Apply defibrillation pads either in sternal/apex or anterior/posterior position
    a. Hands-free defibrillation pads
        1) Follow manufacturer's recommendation of pad placement
        2) Assure pads have good skin contact
        3) Pads should be at least 1 inch (2.5cm) apart
        4) Attach defibrillation pad cable to defibrillator
        5) When performing defibrillation (step #10 below), press the appropriate button
    b. Defibrillation paddles
        1) Appling the paddles to the patient may be done after charging
        2) Electrode jelly or gel defibrillation pads should be used with paddles
        3) Paddles must be in full contact with patient's skin
        4) Place paddles in the sternal/apex position (upper right anterior chest under the clavicle and on the left chest at the 5th intercostal space between the mid-clavicular and anterior axillary lines)
        5) When performing defibrillation (step #10 below), hold paddles firmly in place and apply 25 pounds of pressure on each paddle until the machine discharges
        6) Select energy level after identifying as ventricular fibrillation or pulse ventricular tachycardia
        7) Charge the defibrillator
        8) Start paper recording to document rhythm. Information may be stored on a memory card on some units
        9) Verbally and visually "clear" everyone from the patient.
        10) Deliver defibrillation by pressing the correct button
        11) Resume high quality CPR immediately after defibrillation
        12) Coordinate prompt and repeated defibrillation with CPR and other basic and advanced skills
            a. Oxygen administration
            b. Airway placement
            c. Vascular access
            d. Medication administration

        13) Repeat steps 5 – 11 as needed

B. SYNCHRONIZED CARDIOVERSION

POINTS OF EMPHASIS
- Assess the environment for safety concerns when performing cardioversion (patent clear of fluids/puddles, good adherence of defibrillation pads, etc.)
- Complete patient assessment to determine if patient's instability is due to rapid heart rate.
- Consider administering a sedative prior to performing cardioversion as patient condition allows.
- Prep the area where pads are to be applied by drying the skin, removing debris, minimizing hair, etc.
- Adjust size (gain) or lead being used to ensure QRS is properly 'flagged'.
- Select cardioversion energy per AHA guidelines and manufacturer recommendations for model of defibrillator.
- Many defibrillator units require operator to activate synchronization mode every time. Other units will stay in synchronization mode until they are manually turned off.
- Always verbally and visually 'clear' the patient prior to cardioverting the patient.
- Initiate an IV/IO as soon as possible.
- Unsynchronized cardioversion can be done in an unstable patient when you cannot get the defibrillator to synchronize.

SKILLS
1. Turn the monitor/defibrillator on and check that defibrillation cable is attached to unit.
2. Identify the rhythm as tachycardia and the patient is symptomatic due to tachycardia.
3. Obtain a 12 lead ECG, if able
4. Determine what the rhythm is in order to select the correct energy level
5. Explain the procedure to the patient
6. Apply defibrillation pads either in sternal/apex or anterior/posterior position
   a. Hands-free defibrillator pads
      1) Follow manufacturer's recommendation for pad placement.
      2) Assure pads have good skin contact
      3) Pads should be placed 1 inch (2.5cm) apart
      4) Attach defibrillation pad cable to defibrillator
      5) When performing cardioversion (step #13), press the appropriate button.
   b. Defibrillation paddles
      1) Applying the paddles to the patient may be done after charging
      2) Electrode jelly or gel defibrillation pads should be used with paddles
      3) Paddles must be in full contact with patient's skin
      4) Place paddles in the sternal/apex position (upper right anterior below the clavicle and on the left chest at the 5th intercostal space between the midclavicular and the anterior axillary lines)
      5) When performing cardioversion (step #13), hold the paddles firmly in place and apply 25 pounds of pressure on each paddle until the machine discharges
7. Activate synchronization mode on the defibrillation unit
8. Identify that the QRS is being flagged
9. Select the energy level
10. Charge the defibrillator
11. Start paper recording to document rhythm. Information may be stored on a memory card on some units.
12. Verbally and visually 'clear' everyone from the patient
13. Deliver cardioversion by pressing and holding the appropriate button

SECTION 6 – MEDICATION PREPARATION AND ADMINISTRATION

OBJECTIVES
- To prepare the appropriate delivery device for the purpose of administering medications
- To prepare the appropriate delivery device for the purpose of administering fluids
- To administer medication enteral and parenteral routes

POINTS OF EMPHASIS
- Use appropriate body substance isolation precautions
- Medication must be administered in compliance with local protocols and medical direction
- A comprehensive assessment must be performed on all patients to whom medications will be administered to determine:
  - Indication for medication
  - Contraindication(s) for medication
  - Appropriate dose for patient
  - Response to medication
- All skills in this section assume the patient is being provided with supplemental oxygen as appropriate
- Before administering any medication, always be certain you have:
  - The right patient
  - The right medication
  - The right dose
  - The right time
  - The right route
  - The right documentation
- Prior to medication preparation and delivery, inspect the medication to insure it:
  - Contains the correct medication
  - Contains the correct dose
  - Has not expired
  - Has not been contaminated in any manner. Non-intact packaging may indicate loss of sterility
- Documentation should include (per local protocol):
  - Medication
  - Dose delivered
  - Route
  - Site/method
  - Time given
  - Physician ordering medication
  - EMS person delivering medication
- Generally rectal administration is contraindicated in the presence of active rectal bleeding, diarrhea and low platelet count.

I. ENTERAL ROUTES: ORAL, SUBLINGUAL, BUCCAL, GASTRIC TUBE, AND RECTAL MEDICATIONS

A. PREPARATION OF ORAL, SUNLINGUAL, BUCCAL, RECTAL, AND GASTRIC MEDICATIONS
  1. Tablets (Oral)
     a. Inspect the medication
     b. Shake out the proper number of tablets to obtain the proper dose

  c. Recheck the label for proper medication and dosage information
  d. Give directions to patient for medication administration
  e. The medication is now ready to be administered
 2. Sublingual spray (Under the tongue)
  a. Inspect the medication
  b. Give directions to patient for medication administration
  c. The medication is now ready to be administered
 3. Buccal (between cheek and gum):
  a. Inspect the medication
  b. Buccal medication may be applied to a tongue depressor for administration
  c. Give directions to patient for medication administration
  d. The medication is now ready to be administered
 4. Gastric Tube
  a. Inspect medication
   1) Liquid form: Preferred type of medication. Measure prescribed dose.
   2) Tablet: Crush pill into fine powder (enteric coated and time released tablets should not be crushed) Mix with at least 30 ml of water. Assure that particles are dissolved in solution.
  b. Draw 30 ml of water to flush the tube after medication administration
  c. Re-check the label for proper medication and dosage information.
  d. The medication is now ready to be administered
 5. Rectal
  a. Inspect the medication
  b. Prepare the medication as needed
   1) Remove packaging
   2) Lubricate syringe tip or suppository
   3) A large bore IV catheter (without the needle, ouch!) can be attached to the syringe for liquid medication administration
  c. Re-check the label for proper medication and dosage information
  d. The medication is now ready to be administered

B. ADMINISTRATION OF ORAL, SUBLINGUAL, AND BUCCAL MEDICATIONS
 1. Prepare medication as previously described in this section
 2. Recheck medication label for the rights
 3. Explain procedure to the patient:
  a. Oral: Swallow the medication with a small amount of water
  b. Chewed: Chew the medication and do not swallow for about 10 seconds
  c. Sublingual: Place the medication under the tongue and do not swallow for 10 seconds
  d. Sublingual spray: Spray on or under the tongue; be careful the patient does not inhale medication
  e. Buccal: Apply medication between patient's cheek and gum
 4. Give the medication to the patient to take or place medication in the patient's mouth
 5. Assure the medication is swallowed, chewed or dissolved
 6. Document medication administration
 7. Provide an ongoing assessment of your patient to identify any effects of the medication

C. ADMINISTRATION OF GASTRIC TUBE MEDICATIONS
 1. Re-check the six rights
 2. Inspect the medication. Assure that it is in liquid form and particles are dissolved in solution
 3. Place patient in a high-Fowler position, unless contraindicated by patient's condition
 4. Explain the procedure to the patient

5. Verify proper placement of the gastric tube by aspirating for gastric contents or by auscultating over the gastric area while injecting a bolus of air
6. Remove the plunger from syringe to be used for medication administration
7. Insert syringe into gastric tube or medication port
8. Pour medication into syringe. Medication should flow by gravity. If it does not, you can:
    a. Raise the syringe height
    b. Reposition the patient
    c. If the above steps do not work, replace the plunger and give a gentle push to facilitate flow.
9. Once the medication administration is complete, flush the gastric tube with 15 ml water
10. Reposition the patient, as needed.

D. ADMINISTERING RECTAL MEDICATIONS
1. Recheck the six rights
2. Inspect the medication
3. Explain rectal procedure to the patient
4. Remove clothing from the waist down so rectum is accessible taking care to provide patient privacy
5. Position the patient
    a. Assist patient into a lateral recumbent position (left side) with the top leg flexed forward
    b. If unable to position patient on side, other positions are acceptable Having one or both patient's legs flexed will facilitate medication administration
6. Recheck medication and lubricate
    a. Suppository: Lubricate rounded end with water soluble lubricant
    b. Syringe: Lubricate tip of syringe with water soluble lubricant
7. Instruct patient to take slow, deep breaths through the mouth and relax anal sphincter
8. Retract patient's buttocks and give medications
    c. a. Suppository: With gloved finger, insert suppository gently through the anus, past the internal sphincter (about 4 inches (10 cm) for adults, 3 inches (7.5 cm) for children, 2 inches (5 cm) for infants)
    d. Syringe: Insert syringe tip gently through anus gently to a depth as indicated in "a" above and gently depress the plunger.
9. Keep finger or syringe in the rectum for about 3 seconds to ensure that medication will not come out.
10. Withdraw finger or syringe and wipe excess lubricant from anal area
11. For best results the patient should remain on their side for 5-10 minutes.

II. INHALED MEDICATIONS

POINTS OF EMPHASIS
- Follow manufacturer's recommendation for liter flow and assembly of equipment.
- Many IM/IV medications can be given via the intranasal route; follow local protocols.
- Only select medications that can be administered via endotracheal route.
- Needles should be removed for medication administration via ETT to prevent accidental puncture of the ETT or loss of needle in the ETT.

A. PREPARATION OF INHALED MEDICATIONS
1. Metered Dose Inhaler

        a. Inspect medication
        b. Shake the inhaler canister vigorously
        c. Wait 1-2 minutes between inhalations; shake canister before each inhalation
    2. Nebulizer
        a. Select a nebulizer delivery method based on the patient's ability to hold the device and coordinate inhalation and breathing technique.
            1) If using the hand-held delivery, attach the reservoir hose and mouthpiece to opposite ends of the "T".
            2) If using a mask delivery, use a nebulizer mask or remove reservoir bag and one-way valves from a non-rebreather mask.
        b. Assemble the medication cup by screwing the top and bottom sections together. Most nebulizers must be kept upright to avoid spilling medication.
        c. Inspect the medication
        d. Place the ordered dose of medication(s) into the medication cup and attach it to the bottom of the "T" fitting or mask.
        e. Attach the oxygen tubing to the inlet port of the medication cup. Attach the other end to an oxygen source capable of delivering 6-8 liters flow.
        f. Turn on oxygen and adjust flow for best results.
    3. Intranasal
        a. Draw up medication to be given in a syringe (se IM/IV medication preparation section).
            1) Maximum volume per nostril is 1 ml.
            2) Add 0.1 ml to dose calculation to account for dead space in atomizer
        b. Attach the atomizer delivery device to syringe (remove needle if one is present)
    4. Endotracheal
        a. Draw up medication to be given in a 10 ml syringe (see IM/IV medication preparation section)
            1) ETT dose is usually 2-2.5 times the IV dose
            2) Add sterile water or saline to make 10 ml

B. ADMINISTRATION OF INHALED MEDICATIONS
    1. Recheck six rights
    2. Metered dose inhaler
        a. Inspect the medication
        b. Verify the inhaler belongs to the patient
        c. Shake the container vigorously
        d. Explain the procedure to the patient
            1) Forcibly exhale
            2) Place lips around the inhaler
            3) Activate inhaler while inhaling
            4) Hold breath as long as comfortably able
        e. Remove supplemental oxygen from the patient if needed for medication administration
        f. Assist with medication administration if needed
        g. Replace the oxygen and encourage the patient to breathe deeply
        h. Repeat steps c-g to obtain ordered dosage(s). Wait 1-2 minutes between inhalations
    3. Nebulizer
        a. Assemble nebulizer delivery device as previously described in this section
        b. Explain procedure to patient
            1) Seal lip around the mouthpiece of the hand-held nebulizer or place mask on patient

            2) Take slow breaths and inhale as deeply as possible
            3) Hold breaths as long as comfortably able, up to 10 seconds
            4) Continue until medication is gone; there is no misting
        c. Remove supplemental oxygen from patient
        d. Start nebulizer with oxygen at 6-8 lpm – adjust until it makes a fine mist
        e. Encourage patient to take slow, deep breaths until the medicine is gone from the medication cup. As the medication is administered and the level drops in the medication cup, the cup may need to be tapped to deliver all the medication.
        f. Replace supplemental oxygen when the treatment is completed
    4. Intranasal
        a. Explain procedure to patient
        b. Place atomizer in nostril
        c. Depress plunger quickly to administer medication
        d. If needed, switch nostrils to administer remaining dose if over than 1 ml
        e. Remove atomizer from nostril
        f. If patient sneezes, medication does not have to be repeated
    5. Endotracheal
        a. Pre-oxygenate the patient with a bag valve device prior to medication delivery
        b. Remove bag valve device and instill medication into the ETT
        c. Distribute medication with positive pressure ventilations prior to resuming normal ventilations with the bag valve device.

III. TOPICAL MEDICATIONS

POINTS OF EMPHASIS
- Application sites for topical medications
    - Avoid hairy areas or scar tissue
    - Preferred areas are chest, back, upper arms, or legs
    - Some patches identify placement location

A. PREPARATION OF TOPICAL MEDICATIONS
1. Nitroglycerine ointment
    a. Inspect medication
    b. Date, time and initial paper guide
    c. apply desired inches of ointment on paper guide
    d. Re-check the label for proper medication and dosage information
    e. Medication is now ready to administer
2. Transdermal Patch
    a. Inspect medication
    b. Using a soft-tip or felt pen, write date, time and your initials on the outer side of the patch (or overlay, if provided)
    c. Re-check the label for proper medication and dosage information
    d. Medication is now ready to be administered

B. ADMINISTRATION OF TOPICAL MEDICATIONS
1. Re-check six rights
2. Nitroglycerine ointment
    a. Remove previous dose paper and wipe off residual medication

b. Apply ointment to skin surface by placing paper measuring guide (with medication towards patient's skin)

  c. Do not rub or massage ointment into the skin

  d. Date, time, and initial paper (maybe done prior to application)

  e. Secure ointment and paper with a transparent dressing or tape

 3. Transdermal Patch

  a. Remove old patches before applying a new patch and wipe off residual medication

  b. Fold old patch in half with sticky sides together prior to disposal

  c. Re-check medication and dose

  d. Select clean, dry area of body. Site should be different from location of old patches

  e. Apply patch to the skin by holding it by the edge and not touching adhesive edges

  f. Press firmly with the palm of one hand for 10 seconds and ensure the patch sticks well around the edges

  g. Apply overlay, if provided with patch

IV. INJECTABLE MEDICATIONS

POINTS OF EMPHASIS

- Maintain sterility of needles and medication for injections
- Utilize safety engineered devices to minimize risk of needle sticks (mandatory except for auto-injectors)
- Identify distal connection type for syringes and IV tubing ('luer lock' vs. 'slip' connection)
- Always ensure that all sharps are properly disposed of in a timely manner in an approved sharps disposal container
- Route of administration and size of the patient are used to determine the appropriate size needle
  - A 23- to 25-gauge, 5/8-inch-long needle is appropriate for subcutaneous injections.
  - The needle gauge for I.M. injections should be larger to accommodate viscous solutions and suspension. Recommend 21G to 23G needles 1" to 2" in length
  - As a rule of thumb, a 200 pound (90 kg) patient requires a longer needle (i.e., 2" or 5 cm) for injection; a 100 lb (45 kg) patient will require a 1 ¼ to 1 ½" needle.
- Pre-filled systems may have an air bubble that will need to be purged prior to medication administration
- When drawing up medication from a vial or ampule, draw up a little extra that can be wasted when purging air bubbles
- Assure the proposed site for injection is free of inflammation, swelling, infection and any skin lesions
- Never recap used needles
- Allow alcohol to dry for 30 seconds for bacteria to be killed and to minimize discomfort of injection
- Prior to injection, tell the patient that they will feel a poke.
- If blood is present when aspirating, withdraw the needle and discard the medication. Start over with new medication and a new site

 A. PREPARATION OF INJECTABLE MEDICATIONS SYRINGE AND VIAL

  1. Inspect the medication
  2. Select an appropriate size syringe for the medication to be delivered
  3. Remove the protective "flip-off" cap from the top of the vial
  4. Wipe the rubber stopper with an alcohol prep or other suitable antiseptic swab
  5. If reconstituting a medication:

a. Pierce the center of the medication vial's stopper with the needle on the syringe of diluting solution
   b. Inject diluting solution
   c. Remove the needle/syringe from the vial
   d. Gently shake the vial to assure the medication dissolves
   e. Continue with drawing up the medication with a new needle and syringe
6. If drawing a medication or diluting solution from a vial:
   a. Draw up the same volume of air as the volume to be withdrawn
   b. Pierce the center of the vial's stopper with the needle on the syringe
   c. Inject air
   d. Holding the vial upside down in one hand and being careful to keep the end of the needle within the fluid level of the vial, pull back gently on the plunger to draw the medication or diluting solution into the syringe
   e. Withdraw the needle and syringe from the vial
7. Replace the needle with an appropriate size safety engineered needle for subcutaneous or IM injections
   a. For patient comfort, change the needle prior to injection. Most needles have a fine silicone coating to facilitate easy entry into muscle mass which may be lost when drawing up medication through the rubber stopper.
   b. Literature has shown that some rubber stoppers contain trace amounts of latex that may cause a sensitivity reaction.
   c. Common practice is to use a larger diameter needle to draw the medication, and a smaller diameter to inject the medication.
8. With the needle pointing upward, gently tap the syringe to move any air bubbles to the top.
9. Gently depress the plunger of the syringe until air is expelled and only the desired amount of medication remains in the syringe
10. The medication is now ready to be delivered

SYRINGE AND AMPULE
1. Inspect the medication
2. Select a syringe of appropriate size for the volume of medication to be delivered
3. Select a filter needle of appropriate size and length to withdraw the medication and attach to the syringe
4. Hold the ampule upright and gently "flick" it to move any medication trapped in the head of the ampule to the base
5. Wipe the area between the head and base of the ampule with an alcohol prep or other suitable antiseptic swab
6. Once the medication is removed from the head of the ampule, open the ampule by holding the ampule at arm's length and break by snapping the head towards you.
   a. Use a commercially available device or a gauze square to grasp the head of the ampule and break the head from the base
   b. If the ampule fails to break cleanly and glass shards can be observed, dispose of the ampule and replace with another.
7. Using the filter needle and syringe withdraw medication for administration. Discard any remaining medication and properly dispose of both portions of the ampule in a sharps container
8. Remove the filter needle used to withdraw the medication from the ampule and properly dispose of the filter needle in an sharps container
9. Replace the filter needle with an appropriate size safety engineered needle for subcutaneous or IM injections

10. With the needle pointing upward, gently tap the syringe to move any air bubbles to the top of the syringe
11. Gently depress the plunger of the syringe until air is expelled and only the desired amount of medication remains in the syringe
12. The medication is now ready to be delivered

PRE-LOADED SYRINGES
1. Pre-filled Systems
    a. Inspect the medication
    b. Remove the protective caps from the medication cartridge and the barrel of the syringe assembly
    c. Insert the medication cartridge into the barrel assembly and rotate clockwise until the medication cartridge is secure in the barrel. The medication cartridge is now the plunger
    d. With the unit now fully assembled, remove the protector from the distal tip and gently depress the plunger until air is expelled and only the desired amount of medication remains in the syringe
    e. Attach an appropriate size safety engineered needle for subcutaneous or IM injections
    f. The medication is now ready to be delivered
2. Syringe Cartridge Systems (e.g. Carpuject and Tubex)
    a. Inspect the medication cartridge
    b. Insert and secure the syringe cartridge into the cartridge holder following the manufacturer's directions
    c. Attach an appropriate size safety engineered needle for subcutaneous or IM injections
    d. With the unit now fully assembled, remove the protector from the distal tip and gently depress the plunger of the syringe until air is expelled and only the desired amount of medication remains in the syringe
    e. The medication is now ready to be delivered
3. Auto-injector systems
    a. Inspect the medication
    b. Remove the safety cap only after placing the device against the previously prepared injection site
    c. The medication is now ready to be administered
B. ADMINISTRATION OF INJECTABLE MEDICATIONS INTRAMUSCULAR INJECTION
    1. Prepare medication as previously described in this section
    2. Recheck medication label for the rights
    3. Ensure the correct size safety needle is attached for administration route (not applicable for auto-injector)
    4. Select an injection site
        a. Deltoid
        b. Vastus lateralis (lateral thigh)
    5. After selecting the injection site, gently tap it to stimulate the nerve endings which will minimize pain when the needle is inserted. Using the stretch technique may accomplish this also
    6. Cleanse the injection site with an alcohol prep or other suitable antiseptic swab in an outward circular motion for about 2 inches
    7. Hold the syringe in dominant hand and remove the needle cover
    8. Stabilize the injection site with your non-dominant hand using:
        a. "Pinch" technique
        b. Stretch technique

9. Holding the syringe like a dart, quickly but not forcefully, insert the needle into the injection site at a 90 degree angle until the proper depth is reached
10. Release the skin while continuing to hold the syringe in place with the dominant hand
11. Grasp the plunger with one hand and the barrel of the device with the other. Pull back (aspirate) slightly on the plunger and wait five seconds
12. If no blood aspirates into the syringe, proceed with the injection. Slowly depress the plunger to administer the injection (10 seconds per mL)
13. Once the medication has been administered, wait ten seconds, then withdraw the needle using appropriate safety features and/or activating the needle safety engineering device
14. Cover the injection site with an alcohol or gauze pad and apply gentle pressure to the area to help reduce pain and improve absorption
15. Properly dispose of the syringe and needle assembly in an appropriate sharps container
16. Place a bandage over the injection site

AUTO-INJECTOR

1. Prepare medication as previously described in this section
2. Recheck medication label for the rights
3. Select the vastus lateralis (lateral thigh) injection site
4. Cleanse the injection site with an alcohol prep or other suitable antiseptic swab in an outward circular motion for about 2 inches
5. Grasp the auto-injector by wrapping fist around the unit, Never place your thumb or finger over the ends of the auto-injector
6. Place dispensing end of auto-injector against the prepared site on the lateral thigh at a 90 degree angle
7. Remove the protective cap
8. Stabilize the patient's leg to prevent pulling away
9. Apply a gentle pressure against leg with auto-injector until it clicks
10. Hold in place for 10 seconds before removing auto-injector
11. Properly dispose of the auto-injector in an appropriate sharps container
12. Place a bandage over the injection site

SUBCUTANEOUS INJECTION

1. Prepare medication as previously described in this section
2. Recheck six rights
3. Insure the correct size safety needle is attached for administration route (not applicable for auto-injector)
4. Select an injection site
5. Cleanse the injection site with alcohol prep or other suitable antiseptic swab in an outward circular motion for about 2 inches
6. Hold the syringe in dominant hand and remove the needle cover
7. Stabilize the injection site with your non-dominant hand using the "pinch" technique
8. Holding the syringe like a dart, quickly but not forcefully, insert the needle into the injection site at a 45-90 degree angle until the proper depth is reached
9. Release the skin while continuing to hold the syringe in place with the dominant hand
10. Slowly depress the plunger to administer the injection (10 seconds per mL)
11. Once the medication has been administered, wait ten seconds, then withdraw the needle using appropriate safety features
12. Cover the injection site with an alcohol or gauze pad and put gentle pressure on the area to help reduce pain and improve absorption

13. Properly dispose of the syringe and needle assembly in an appropriate sharps container
14. Place a bandage over the injection site

INTRAVENOUS BOLUS MEDICATIONS (IVP) - Assumes a patent IV is present
1. Prepare medication as previously described in this section
2. Recheck six rights
3. Insure the correct size safety needle is attached for administration route (not applicable for auto-injector)
4. Use alcohol prep or other suitable antiseptic swab to wipe the surface of the IV tubing med-port closest to the patient
5. Remove the protective cap from the syringe
6. Connect the syringe to the prepared med-port by:
    a. Twisting clockwise for luer lock connections
    b. Inserting blunt cannula for ports designed for this safety device
    c. Inserting needle through self-sealing ports designed for needle puncture
7. Kink off the IV tubing between the selected med-port and the IV solution bag
8. Inject the medication at the proper rate
9. Disconnect syringe from med-port
10. Following injection of the medication, flush the IV tubing
    a. Bolus flush by syringe
    b. Open flow of IV
11. Properly dispose of the syringe and needle assembly in an appropriate sharps container

V. INTRAVENOUS / INTRAOSSEOUS ADMINISTRATION AND CARE

POINTS OF EMPHASIS
- Maintain sterility of needles, ends of IV tubing and medication for injections
- An intraosseous (IO) line is used the same as an intravenous (IV) line for fluid and medication administration
- Utilize safety engineered devices to minimize risk of needle sticks (mandatory)
- Always insure that all sharps are properly disposed of in a timely manner in an approved sharps disposal container.
- Assure the proposed site for cannulation is free of inflammation, swelling, infection and any skin lesions
- Never recap used needles
- Allow alcohol to dry for 0 seconds for bacteria to be killed and minimize discomfort during insertion
- Whenever possible, the IV bag should be hung vertically to facilitate preparation.
- If too much fluid enters the drip chamber, invert the bag and drip chamber and squeeze some of the fluid back into the bag
- If tape is used, it should be torn to length prior to beginning the preparation procedures
- Taping methods and commercial securing devices are available. Follow local protocol.
- For IO insertion
    - Landmarking correctly helps avoid piercing the growth plate. If unable to landmark, choose a different site.
    - A –way stopcock is optional and can be used at the hub or distal end of the extension tubing.

- Aspiration of cloudy fluid is optional since lack of cloudy aspirate is not uncommon and does not indicate improper placement.
- If the IO does not flow, apply pressure to the IV bag by squeezing it. If this works, place a pressure device on the IV bag.

A. IV ADMINISTRATION SET PREPARATION
1. Select the appropriate solution
    a. Inspect the solution; A slight amount of moisture inside the outer bag is normal and not cause for concern
    b. Open outer packaging by tearing pre-cut slit at either end of the bag
        1) Recheck clarity
2. Select an appropriate IV administration set
3. Open the administration set
    a. Check to be certain the end caps that preserve the sterile field of the administration set remain in place
    b. Uncoil the tubing in preparation for spiking the IV bag
    c. If adjunct devices such as extensions or flow meters are to be used, they should be opened and attached to the administration set at this time
4. Move the flow control clamp to a convenient location and close off the IV tubing by:
    a. Rotating the control knob (roller clamp)
    b. Sliding the clamp (slide clamp)
    c. Pinching the clamp (pinch clamp)
5. Spike the IV bag
    a. Method one
        1) If not previously done, hang the IV bag with the tail ports extending downward
        2) Grasp the IV port just above the plastic tab. With the other hand, pull the plastic tab from the port. Be careful to maintain sterility of the port
        3) Remove the protective cap from the IV tubing spike being careful to protect the sterile field
        4) Insert the IV tubing spike into the IV port by pushing and twisting the spike until it punctures the seal of the port
        5) Squeeze the drip chamber to fill it approximately half full of fluid
    b. Method two
        1) Holding the IV bag at its base, invert the bag so the tail ports extend upward
        2) While continuing to hold the IV bag, grasp its IV port just below the plastic tab. With the other hand, pull the plastic tab from the port. Be careful to maintain sterility of the port
        3) Remove the protective cap from the IV tubing spike being careful to protect the sterile field
        4) Insert the IV tubing spike into the IV port by pushing and twisting the spike until it punctures the seal of the port
        5) Invert the bag so it is in an upright position and hang the IV bag
        6) Squeeze the drip chamber to fill it approximately half full of fluid
6. Place the end of the tubing in a convenient location while preserving sterility by keeping protective cap in place
7. Open the flow control clamp and allow the IV fluid to completely fill the line. It is often necessary to invert and "flick" med-ports with your fingers to remove larger air bubbles

8. Once the line is completely filled with fluid, and larger air bubbles removed, close the flow clamp and place the "primed" line in position for use

B. INITIATING VENOUS ACCESS
1. Prepare IV administration system as previously described in this section
2. Prepare the necessary equipment and supplies
    a. Sharps container
    b. Tape and/or commercially available device for securing the IV
    c. Alcohol prep pads or other suitable antiseptic swab
    d. Gauze pads
    e. Site dressing
    f. Tourniquet (latex free)
    g. Catheter(s)
    h. Band-aid
3. Select a venipuncture area (hand, wrist, forearm or antecubital space)
4. Apply a venous tourniquet approximately 4 to 8 inches above the selected area
5. Select a vein for cannulation and cleanse the intended venipuncture site with an alcohol prep or other suitable antiseptic swab in an outward circular motion for at least 2 inches
6. Based on the intent of the IV and the size of the vein selected, choose an appropriate size IV catheter
7. Remove the catheter from its packaging and the protective plastic sheath
8. Being careful to maintain the sterility of the needle and catheter, visually inspect the end of each for any defects, such as burred edges
9. Slightly twist the catheter on the needle to insure the catheter moves freely on the needle (optional step)
10. Grasp the patient's extremity near the area where the IV will be started using your non-dominant hand in order to stabilize the vein at the venipuncture site. This may be accomplished by:
    a. Pulling traction distal
    b. Holding extremity circumferentially so area is taut
11. Insure the bevel of the needle is facing upward in relation to the patient's skin
12. Holding the catheter assembly with fingers of your dominant hand, and in such a manner as to be able to visualize the flash chamber, approach the injection site with the needle held at approximately a 15 – 20 degree angle
13. Inform the patient they will feel a slight "pinch" as the needle enters their skin
14. While continuing to apply traction to the skin to hold the vein steady, quickly, but carefully, enter the skin with the needle and continue until the needle tip is against the wall of the vein itself. Maintain traction and vein stabilization until catheter is in the lumen of the vein
15. Slowly advance the needle through the vein wall and into the lumen of the vein
    a. A "pop" may be felt as the needle enters the vein.
    b. The flash chamber should fill with blood when entering the vein.
        1) Smaller catheters will be slower to have a flash
        2) Patients with poor perfusion may not have a significant flash
16. Once you have entered the vein, continue to advance the needle and catheter assembly slightly (0.5 cm further) so the tip of the catheter enters the vein
17. When the catheter tip is within the lumen of the vein, slowly advance the catheter along the needle until the hub meets the patient's skin. Slide the catheter while holding the needle steady

18. After the catheter has been threaded into the vein, slightly pull back the needle from the catheter, but DO NOT withdraw it completely
19. If not drawing blood via the IV catheter, release the tourniquet. If blood draws are to be made using the IV catheter, leave the tourniquet in place and obtain blood samples before releasing tourniquet
20. Palpate the end of the catheter beneath the patient's skin and occlude the vein just proximal to the end of the catheter with direct pressure
21. Remove the needle and activate any safety features before disposing of it in an approved sharps container
22. With your free hand, remove the protective cap from the end of the IV tubing and attach it to the catheter hub, making sure not to push the catheter further in or pull it out
23. Open the IV flow clamp and observe the flow of fluid into the drip chamber
    a. If the IV does not flow:
        1) Insure the tourniquet has been released
        2) Carefully withdraw the catheter slightly while observing the drip chamber since the tip may be occluded by a valve or the side of the vein
        3) Determine if the IV is positional and troubleshoot as necessary
        4) Begin the process anew using another site
    b. With the IV running, and before securing the IV catheter in place, inspect the venipuncture site for signs of infiltration
    c. If an IV cannot be made to flow properly or infiltration is observed, discontinue the IV immediately
24. If the IV is observed to flow properly:
    a. Using a gauze pad or alcohol prep pad as necessary, wipe away any fluid or blood that may be present in order to dry the site sufficiently that tape will adhere
    b. Secure the IV and the IV tubing in place; cover insertion site with a sterile dressing or commercially available device
25. Secure the patient's extremity as appropriate to maintain flow
26. Adjust the flow rate by closing flow clamp or other flow-metering device to the appropriate setting
27. Continue to monitor the patient for:
    a. Signs of a fluid overload
    b. Other complications resulting from the IV
    c. Appropriate flow rate
    d. Infiltration
28. Continue to monitor the IV to insure appropriate flow rate is maintained and the venipuncture does not infiltrate

C. CHANGING THE SOLUTION BAG OF AN ESTABLISHED IV
1. Select and inspect the IV solution
2. Open outer packaging by tearing pre-cut slit at either end of the bag
3. Shut off the flow clamp on the nearly empty IV bag to prevent air from entering the IV tubing as the solution bag is being changed
4. Invert the nearly empty bag to prevent any remaining fluid from running out, and remove the IV tubing spike from the bag
    a. Use extreme care to ensure the IV tubing spike does not touch anything to contaminate the sterile field
    b. Follow one of the methods previously described in this section to puncture the bag

c. Discard the used solution bag after noting the approximate amount of any remaining fluid
4. Reestablish the IV flow rate

D. INTRAVENOUS PIGGYBACK (IVPB) MEDICATION (assumes a patient primary IV is infusing)
1. Inspect the medication or premixed IV solution
2. If using premixed medicated IV solution, the medication is now ready to be administered.
3. If mixing the piggyback IV bag:
    a. Draw up the correct amount of the medication into a syringe as described above.
    b. Select the appropriate IV solution and size for the piggyback.
    c. Cleanse the medication port on the IV line.
    d. Insert the needle into the medication port
    e. Depress the plunger to inject the medication into the piggyback IV bag
    f. Withdraw needle and discard into a sharps container
    g. Mix medication thoroughly in piggyback IV bag.
    h. Label piggyback IV bag with:
        1) Name of the medication
        2) Amount of medication
        3) Date and time medication added
        4) Name and initials of preparer
    i. Calculate the dose mg/ml and gtt/min that is needed
    j. Select the appropriate IV tubing based on above calculations
    k. Spike the piggyback IV bag and flush the tubing
    l. Piggyback medication is now ready to be administered
    m. Re-check the six rights and infusion calculations for dose/ml and gtt/min that is needed.
    n. Clean the medication port of the primary IV set. Use one closest to patient.
    o. Connect the piggyback IV tubing to the prepared medication port.
    p. Shut off primary IV tubing flow to ensure the piggyback fluid is flowing to the patient.
    q. Open the flow rate clamp on the piggyback IV tubing and adjust the flow to the desired rate.
    r. Continue to monitor the patient for:
        1) Desired effects and side effects of the IVPB medication
        2) Other complications resulting from the IV
        3) Appropriate flow rate
        4) Infiltration
    s. Continue monitoring the IVPB to ensure flow rate is maintained and the venipuncture does not infiltrate.
    t. When stopping the IVPB medication, shut off the flow control clamp on the IVPB tubing. Open primary IV tubing using its flow control clamp and adjust rate of primary solution.

E. DISCONTINUING AN IV
1. Prepare the necessary materials
    a. Gauze square(s)
    b. Tape
    c. Band-Aid
    d. Disposal container

2. Close the flow clamp of the IV administration set
3. Gently remove the tape and/or securing device to expose the venipuncture site
4. Cover the venipuncture site with a gauze square and apply gentle pressure as you remove the IV catheter
5. Inspect the catheter to insure it is complete, noting any abnormalities
6. Affix an adhesive bandage that will continue to apply pressure until bleeding has stopped
7. Properly dispose of all materials
8. Monitor venipuncture site for bleeding

F. INITIATING AN INTRAOSSEOUS INFUSION
    1. Prepare IV administration system as previously described.
    2. Prepare the necessary equipment and supplies
        a. Sharps container
        b. Tape or commercial device for securing the IO
        c. Alcohol prep pads
        d. Gauze pads
        e. Site dressing
        f. IO device
        g. Syringe with saline for flush
        h. 3-way cockstop (optional)
    3. Select an intraosseous site as approved by local protocol and identify landmarks
        a. Proximal tibia
            1) Flex the knee slightly to facilitate Landmarking
            2) Palpate the tibial tuberosity, just below the knee
            3) Locate the consistent flat area of bone 2 cm distally and 2 cm medially to the tibial tuberosity.
        b. Distal tibia
            1) Slightly abduct and externally rotate the hip to expose the site
            2) Palpate the medial malleolus
            3) Move your finger about 3 cm proximal and palpate the anterior and posterior boundaries of the tibia
            4) Insertion site is on the flat center aspect of the bone
        c. Proximal Humerus
            1) Position the patient so the arm is adducted (closest to the patient)
                a) Flexed at the elbow with palm against abdomen
                b) With extend arm at side, rotate medially with thumb to the posterior
            2) Slide your thumb up the anterior shaft of the humerus until greater tubercle is noted
            3) Insertion point is approximately 1 cm above the greater tubercle
        d. Sternum
            1) Position the patient to access the sternum
            2) Commercial devices are used for this procedure; follow manufacturer's instruction for landmarking injection site.
            3) Choose the appropriate sized IO needle or device and prepare it for insertion. Some commercial devices require adjustment for insertion depth.
            4) Consider using a local anesthetic prior to needle puncture
            5) Cleanse the site with an alcohol swab in an outward motion for at least 2 inches (5 cm)

6) Stabilize the insertion site with the non-dominant
7) Place the IO needle / device against the insertion site
8) If manual IO is used, it is advanced with a back and forth rotational movement
9) If a commercial device is used, follow manufacturer's directions
10) Once inserted, remove the trocar, IO needle will stand up unsupported
11) Attach a syringe filled with saline to the needle/catheter or the extension set.
12) Inject saline into the bone watching for signs of infiltration. If signs are seen, remove the IO needle from the bone and apply gentle pressure to the site.
13) When IO placement is verified, remove syringe and attach the IV line
14) Open the IV flow clamp and observe flow of IV solution in drip chamber
15) Secure the IO needle/catheter, supporting it as needed. Extremity may need to be secured to minimize movement.
16) Cover the insertion site with a sterile dressing or commercial device
17) Secure the patient's extremity as appropriate to maintain flow
18) Adjust the flow rate by closing flow clamp or other flow-metering device to the appropriate setting
19) Continue to monitor the patient for:
 a) Signs of fluid overload
 b) Other complications resulting from IO insertion
 c) Appropriate flow rate
 d) Infiltration
20) Continue to monitor the IO to ensure appropriate flow rate is maintained and the venipuncture does not infiltrate.

SECTION 7 – MANAGEMENT OF SOFT TISSUE INJURIES

OBJECTIVES:
- To control external bleeding.
- To prevent further injury and reduce pain.
- To prevent further wound contamination and reduce the potential of infection.
- To secure dressings through the application of appropriate bandaging techniques.

POINTS OF EMPHASIS:
- Consider MOI for other injuries
- Use appropriate body substance isolation precautions
- Expose the wound site to determine the extent of injury
- Control bleeding by using the following techniques as needed: direct pressure, pressure dressing, elevation, pressure points, cold application and tourniquet
- Use sterile dressings
- Cover the entire wound site with the sterile surface of the dressing
- Apply bandage snugly, making certain not to cut off circulation distal to injury site
- Secure the dressing(s) with roller gauze or cravats applying gentle, even pressure over the wound site
- Consider shock and prevent/treat as appropriate: oxygen, patient positioning, maintenance of body temperature
- CMS should be checked frequently and bandaging adjusted to maintain a pulse if necessary

I. BLEEDING CONTROL

POINTS OF EMPHASIS
- Must be addressed and controlled in the primary assessment
- Bleeding control is part of the "C" in the "ABC's".
- Do not let spinal immobilization interfere with bleeding control. Do not hide an uncontrollable wound with a C-collar.
- Direct pressure with a gloved finger or hand is the most effective means of bleeding control; even larger wounds may have a single point of maximal bleeding.
- Soaked bandages indicate uncontrolled bleeding.
- Hemostatic agents are intended for use by EMT, AEMT, and Paramedic level personnel.

SKILLS:
1. Expose the injuries
2. Direct pressure is the mainstay of bleeding control
    a. Apply direct pressure as close as possible to actual source of bleeding (i.e. fingertip on the end of a bleeding vessel)
        1) Place tip of finger on the end of a cut artery
        2) Pinch the edges of a wound, particularly those on the scalp, between the fingers and thumb.
    b. Use pressure dressings, ensuring the bandages are not so thick as to prohibit monitoring the site.
3. If bleeding continues, remove bandages and look for the source of the bleed to provide re-directed, well-aimed, direct pressure.

4. If bleeding continues, a tourniquet should be used.
5. Large wounds without an identifiable point source should be packed with bandages and broad pressure applied with continued monitoring for bleeding control.
6. If air splints are used for direct pressure, ensure the wound can be visualized to monitor bleeding control.
7. Consider use of hemostatic agents or dressings in available.

II. HEAD

POINTS OF EMPHASIS:
- Do not exert point pressure to scalp if underlying fracture is suspected
- Do not pack nose or ear to stop blood or cerebral spinal fluid (CSF) flow
- Use the patient's brow ridge, chin and occipital ridge as necessary to provide natural anchoring points for bandaging
- If the chin is used, monitor the patient carefully for airway problems. Cut bandage and fold flaps up if bandage interferes with airway or causes patient discomfort

SKILLS:

HEAD (side wound)
1. Open dressing to preserve sterile surface
2. Apply sterile surface to wound site and control bleeding
3. Anchor bandage securely under brow and occipital ridges.
4. Cover dressing completely with bandage
5. Exert even pressure over the entire wound site with finished bandage
6. Leave eyes uncovered, leave ears either completely covered or completely uncovered

HEAD (top wound)
1. Open dressing to preserve sterile surface
2. Apply sterile surface to wound site and control bleeding
3. Anchor bandage securely under brow and occipital ridges.
4. Bring bandage over dressing and under chin and tighten down over dressing
5. Cover dressing completely with bandage, exert even pressure over the entire wound site with finished bandage.
6. Anchor bandage securely by making additional wraps around head, securing under brow ridge and occipital ridge
7. Cut bandage under chin and fold ends up if it interferes with the airway
8. Make last few turns around brow, overlapping folded section

III. EYE

POINTS OF EMPHASIS:
- If areas around eye are lacerated but the eyeball is not involved, use direct pressure to control bleeding
- If eyeball injury is suspected, close eye and apply loose dressing
- If chemical burn is involved, irrigate eye with normal saline continuously
- If thermal burns are involved, apply dressing moistened with sterile saline solution

- If light burns are involved, cover eyes with moist, lightproof pads
- Cover both eyes when injury occurs as consensual eye movement may cause further injury
- Never touch the globe or the penetrating object with your hand
- The finished bandage should hold the eye and/or penetrating object in place
- Maintain verbal and physical contact with the patient as you explain your actions
- Always irrigate from the bridge of the nose outward in order to avoid infecting or contaminating the uninjured eye

SKILLS:

EYE INJURY – Non-penetrating
1. Have patient close eyes
2. Apply sterile surface of dressing to injury(ies)
3. Secure bandage around head, anchoring under occipital ridge
   a. Bandage snugly if eyeball is uninjured
   b. Bandage loosely if injury to the globe is suspected
4. Cover both eyes with finished bandage; do not occlude mouth or nose
5. Restrain patient's hands to keep from touching the eye area as needed

EYE INJURY – Penetrating
1. Surround injured eye with sterile padding
2. If penetrating object, cut hole in end of cup just large enough for object to pass through
3. Place cup or cone over eye, resting it on pads, but do not touch the eye
4. Secure the cup/cone to head with bandage wrapped around cup and then around head anchoring on occipital ridge
5. Wrap bandage to cover uninjured eye, leaving the nose and mouth exposed
6. Restrain patient's hands as necessary to prevent patient from touching the bandaged area

IV. NECK

POINTS OF EMPHASIS
- Use an occlusive dressing to prevent air embolus from being sucked into jugular vein
- DO NOT use a circumferential bandage around the neck

SKILLS:
1. Place dressing over wound
2. Secure dressing in place by wrapping the bandage over the dressing and over the top of the opposite shoulder, crossing under the axilla and back again to form a figure eight
3. Unless contraindicated, transport patient on left side in moderate Trendelenberg position.

V. TORSO

POINTS OF EMPHASIS
- Chest injuries can be life threatening and must be assessed and treated immediately
- Penetrating objects should be left in place unless they interfere with the patient's ability to breathe or maintain an airway

- Penetrating objects must be removed if CPR is necessary
- All open or penetrating injuries to the chest or abdomen must be sealed with an occlusive dressing
- Large penetrating objects should be shortened to facilitate transport or provide stabilization
- Control bleeding with direct pressure around organs, never on top of them
- Look for multiple entry/exit wounds with any form of penetrating trauma
- Use sterile solution soaked dressings on protruding organs
- Administer high flow oxygen and assist ventilations as appropriate
- Transport patients rapidly to the closest appropriate medical facility
- Consider ALS intercept early where available

SKILLS:

A. OPEN CHEST (SUCKING CHEST)
   1. Immediately apply manual pressure to seal wound after patient forcibly exhales
   2. Apply and secure an occlusive dressing,
   3. Auscultate for breath sounds
   4. Closely monitor patient for signs of deterioration

B. PENETRATING OBJECT
   1. Stabilize object with hand(s)
   2. If in chest, upper abdomen or neck area , apply occlusive dressing surrounding the base of the object
   3. Stack bulky dressings in alternating layers to stabilize object from all sides
   4. Secure dressings with bandage to control bleeding and immobilize the object
   5. Restrain patient's hands as necessary to prevent patient from removing object
   6. Transport rapidly in position of comfort

C. ABDOMINAL EVISCERATION
   1. Cover exposed or protruding organs with a sterile dressing moistened with sterile saline
   2. Cover with occlusive dressing to prevent moisture loss
   3. Cover with bulky dressings to preserve body warmth
   4. Secure dressings loosely in place
   5. Transport patient in supine or lateral recumbent position with knees flexed

D. SHOULDER

POINTS OF EMPHASIS
- May be accompanied by fractures or dislocations
- Suspect C-spine injury with significant MOI
- Remove patient's jewelry from affected extremity

SKILLS:

   1. Apply sterile dressing to wound and control bleeding with direct pressure
   2. Check CMS distal to injury prior to applying bandages
   3. Position forearm flexed across chest and bring upper arm along line of body

    4. Wrap bandage around body, covering wounded arm and crossing under arm on the uninjured side to secure dressing
    5. Recheck CMS distal to injury

E. AXILLARY

POINTS OF EMPHASIS:
- Dressing of axillary wounds can easily impair circulation. Check CMS often
- Remove patient's jewelry from affected extremity

SKILLS:
   1. Apply sterile surface of dressing to wound and control bleeding with direct pressure
   2. Check CMS distal to injury prior to applying bandages
   3. Add dressings over the first to achieve bulk as necessary
   4. Bandage around injured armpit and shoulder
   5. Position forearm flexed across chest, hand pointing toward opposite shoulder. Recheck CMS
   6. Wrap bandage around body, over outside surface of arm on injured side and under opposite shoulder
   7. Recheck CMS distal to injury

F. EXTERNAL GENITALIA

IMPORTANT POINTS:
- Preserve the patient's privacy
- Expose genitalia only if wound is suspected

SKILLS:
   1. Apply sterile dressing to wound site and control bleeding
   2. Secure the dressing by running a bandage over dressing, between legs and around pelvis.

VI. EXTREMITIES

POINTS OF EMPHASIS
- Remove patient's jewelry from the affected extremity
- Elevate extremity to reduce pain and control bleeding, if circulation is present
- Leave digits exposed whenever possible
- Consider use of splint to restrict movement

SKILLS:

A. HAND
   1. Check CMS
   2. Apply sterile surface of dressing to wound and control bleeding
   3. Place bandage roll or dressing in palm of hand to maintain position of function
   4. Anchor bandage around wrist
   5. Wrap hand to prevent release from position of function
   6. Achieve some restriction of wrist joint movement with bandage

7. Place hand in elevated position
8. Recheck CMS distal to injury

B. AMPUTATION/AVULSION

POINTS OF EMPHASIS
- Save all amputated or avulsed parts. Transport with patient whenever possible
- Follow local protocols as to application of dry or moist dressings.
- Wrap in a sterile dressing.
- Protect in watertight container.
- Keep part(s) cool during transport, but do not allow to freeze.

SKILL:
1. Apply sterile dressing to wound and control bleeding with direct pressure
2. Wrap bandage around circumference of extremity and pass bandage several times across end of stump to achieve pressure over bleeding area, then secure with several additional circumferential turns
3. Keep stump elevated, if possible
4. If partially attached:
    a. Fold skin flap back over wound
    b. Secure with sufficient pressure to control bleeding
    c. Keep partial amputation cool

VII. BURNS

POINTS OF EMPHASIS
- Make certain the scene is safe to enter
- Always take appropriate hazard precautions as well as body substance isolation precautions
- Burns involving the hands, feet, face or genitalia should be considered critical burns
- Any burns associated with respiratory injuries are critical injuries
- Burn patients are especially susceptible to shock (hypoperfusion) and hypothermia.
- Care must be taken to minimize the potential for infection when dealing with burn patients
- Never use any type of ointment, lotion or antiseptic
- Avoid breaking blisters

SKILLS:
A. THERMAL BURNS
1. Stop the burning process as rapidly as possible using water or saline
2. Remove jewelry and any easily removable clothing or debris from the affected area
3. Continually monitor the airway and breathing for signs of airway impairment or respiratory distress
4. Prevent further contamination of the burned area
5. Cover the wound with a clean and dry dressing
6. Treat for shock
7. Transport

B. ELECTRICAL BURNS

1. Do not attempt to remove a patient from the electrical source unless trained to do so
2. Do not touch a patient unless you are certain s/he is no longer in contact with the electrical source
3. If appropriate, and after assuring no electrical threat remains, stop the burning process as rapidly as possible using water or saline
4. Remove jewelry, and any easily removable clothing, or debris from the affected area
5. Continually monitor the airway and breathing for signs of airway impairment or respiratory distress
6. Monitor the patient for signs of cardia impairment or irregularity
7. Prevent further contamination of the burned area
8. Treat any soft tissue injuries or fractures associated with the burn. Look for multiple entry/exit wounds
9. Cover any exposed burned area with a dry, sterile dressing
10. Treat for shock
11. Transport

C. CHEMICAL BURN
1. Always consider the potential impact of hazardous materials. Patient(s) should not be transported until primary decontamination is completed
2. Brush dry powders off prior to flushing
3. Remove jewelry and any easily removable clothing or debris from the affected area
4. Flush the affected areas with large quantities of water or saline
5. Continue flushing the contaminated area(s) during transport
6. Do not contaminate uninjured or unaffected areas while flushing
7. Continually monitor the airway and breathing for signs of airway impairment or respiratory distress
9. Prevent further contamination of the burned area
10. Treat any soft tissue injuries associated with the burn
11. Treat for shock
12. Transport

SECTION 8 – PNEUMATIC ANTI-SHOCK GARMENT

OBJECTIVES:
- To define the indications and contraindications for the use of the pneumatic compression trousers
- To define the manner in which the PASG can be used to stabilize suspected pelvic fractures and apply circumferential pressure to suspected intra-abdominal bleeding accompanied by signs of shock

POINTS OF EMPHASIS:
- PASG may be applied without inflation to any patient having the potential to develop shock. A systolic blood pressure of 90 mm HG or less, associated with signs and symptoms is generally regarded as a prime indicator for inflation. However, protocols vary Inflate the PASG based on protocol
- The only absolute contraindication to inflation is pulmonary edema
- There are relative contraindications to inflation of all three compartments
- Inflation should be only to a level at which shock symptoms subside. Careful and frequent monitoring of the vital signs after inflation is essential
- Do not deflate in the field unless ordered to do so by medical control

NOTE: Extreme circumstances may arise when the PASG may be deflated in the field, but only under authority of Medical Control. (Field deflation is not a generally accepted practice)

SKILLS:

A. INFLATION
1. Assess patient for and record signs/symptoms of shock. If spinal injury is suspected, maintain spinal stabilization
2. Determine and record the patient's blood pressure
3. Leave deflated blood pressure cuff in place on patient
4. Auscultate breath sounds
5. Remove clothing from patient's abdomen and lower extremities
6. Assess patient's abdomen, pelvis and lower extremities for wounds or fractures. Record findings
7. Cover any open wounds with sterile dressings and bandage in place
8. Restore alignment of extremity fractures, if possible
9. Contact medical control, if required by local protocol, for permission to inflate garment. If medical control contact is not required, proceed according to local protocol
10. Open and arrange anti-shock garment
11. Apply anti-shock garment
    a. Method One:
        1) Lift patient's lower extremities and buttocks, sliding the garment beneath the patient
        2) If spine injury is suspected, use orthopedic stretcher, log roll or straddle slide to position patient
    b. Method Two:
        1) Loosely secure all three compartments
        2) One rescuer puts pants over his/her arms from the foot end and grasps the patient's ankles
        3) Other rescuers pull garment onto patient like a pair of trousers
12. Verify that the superior edge of the garment is just inferior to the patient's costal margin

13. Secure garment – legs then abdomen
14. Attach inflation pump lines to garment and open all in-line valves
15. Inflate garment until:
    a. Patient's clinical status improves satisfactorily, or
    b. Velcro fasteners begin to crackle, indicating separation, or
    c. Air escapes from relief valve(s)
16. Close all in-line valves
17. Leave inflation pump attached to garment during movement and transport
18. Reassess and record, immediately and at frequent intervals enroute to the hospital, the patient's:
    a. Blood pressure
    b. Pulse rate
    c. Respiratory status
    d. Level of consciousness

B. PASG DEFLATION PROCEDURE

NOTE: Extreme circumstances may arise when the PASG may be deflated in the field, but only under authority of Medical Control. (Field deflation is not a generally accepted practice)

POINTS OF EMPHASIS
- Deflate the PASG only on the order of a physician who has examined the patient in the emergency department
- Deflate only after appropriate resuscitative and stabilization measures have been accomplished
- Deflate only with direct physician supervision

SKILLS:
1. Assure the patient has functioning IV lines
2. Assess and record the patient's vital signs
3. Gradually deflate the abdominal section of the garment
    a. Monitor blood pressure carefully
    b. For each 4 - 6 mm Hg drop in the patient's blood pressure, stop deflation and infuse fluids until stabilized at baseline level
    c. If blood pressure continues to drop despite infusion, re-inflate garment and reassess resuscitation
4. After abdominal deflation, gradually deflate each leg segment while monitoring blood pressure and resuscitating as above.

SECTION 9 – ORTHOPEDIC TRAUMA

OBJECTIVES:
- To immobilize suspected fractures and /or dislocations by adequate immobilization of skeletal structure distal and proximal to the injury site
- To apply manual stabilization and utilize appropriate splinting techniques
- To determine the presence or absence of circulation, movement and sensation distal to the injury site
- To restore normal circulation distal to injury sites whenever possible and appropriate, with one attempt to align with gentle traction before splinting
- To reduce the potential of further injury to nerves, blood vessels and soft tissue surrounding the injury site
- To reduce hemorrhage and pain at the injury site and thereby reduce and/or minimize the potential of injury related shock

POINTS OF EMPHASIS:
- Control external bleeding, as needed
- Prevent further wound contamination and reduce the potential of subsequent infection by covering open wounds with a sterile dressing
- Assess circulation, movement and sensation (CMS) prior to and following splint application; loosen splint, if necessary, to regain pulse
- Prevent further injury and reduce pain by immobilizing the joint above and below the long bone injury
- Prevent further injury and reduce pain by immobilizing the bone above and below the joint injury
- Remove clothing from affected area prior to splinting
- Pad as appropriate to prevent pressure and discomfort to patient
- Consider application of cold packs to injury site to reduce swelling
- Always consider the Mechanism of Injury (MOI)
- Suspect cervical spine injury with significant MOI
- Consider shock and prevent/treat as appropriate: oxygen, patient positioning, maintenance of body temperature
- Use of commercial splints should be in accordance with manufacturer's directions

I. THORAX

POINTS OF EMPHASIS:
- Provide oxygen and assist ventilations as necessary
- Monitor patient closely for signs and symptoms of a pneumothorax
- Lung sounds should be auscultated before and after application of dressing
- Encourage and facilitate deep breathing
- In injuries involving the shoulder girdle, it is important to immobilize the entire shoulder girdle
- Sling and swath method:
  - Check CMS in the extremity on the injured side
  - Position forearm of the injured side across the chest, hand slightly elevated toward opposite shoulder. Pad voids between arm and chest if needed.
  - Place triangular bandage under and over the arm with point at the elbow and end tied around the neck. Knot should be placed on the side of the neck of the patient.
  - Pin or tie pointed end to form a cup to support elbow
  - Leave fingers exposed to facilitate CMS check

- Wrap wide bandage around injured arm and body as swathe to pull injured shoulder back and secure to body.
- Re-check CMS in extremity on the injured side
- Transport in sitting or semi-sitting position, if patient's condition permits.

SKILLS:

A. RIB INJURIES
1. Position forearm of injured side across chest, hand slightly elevated toward opposite shoulder and secure with roller bandage or sling and swathe
2. If using a sling and swathe, place triangular bandage under and over arm with point at elbow and two ends tied around patient's neck. Knot should be to the side of the neck
3. Pin or tie end to form cup to support elbow
4. Transport in sitting or semi-sitting position, if patient's condition allows

B. FLAIL CHEST
1. Immediately apply manual stabilization of the flail segment
2. Secure the flail segment with a bulky dressing
3. Place patient in the supine position or on injured side while maintaining spinal immobilization as appropriate
4. Provide oxygen and assist ventilations as necessary

COLLAR BONE (CLAVICAL) SHOULDER BLADE AND SHOULDER INJURIES
1 Sling and swathe method.

II. EXTREMITIES

POINTS OF EMPHASIS: (Upper extremities)
- Apply and maintain manual stabilization of the extremity until the splinting process is complete
- Align severely angulated fractures with gentle traction unless resistance is felt
- Do not attempt to replace protruding bone ends into the wound, if present
- Injuries involving joints should be immobilized in the position found
- Make one attempt to restore circulation distal to an injury site
- Avoid applying pressure to the injury site, whenever possible
- Remove jewelry from injured extremities, place hands in position of function
- Transport patient in sitting or semi-sitting position, as patient's condition permits

SKILLS:
A. ARM (Humerus)
1. Check CMS distal to injury site
2. Stabilize manually proximal and distal to injury site
3. First MEDIC will straighten any severe angulation with gentle traction above and below the fracture site
4. Place a rigid splint on the lateral aspect of the arm to maintain alignment and secure in place
5. Apply wrist sling and swathe to the injured arm to hold the arm in place, elevating the hand and immobilizing the shoulder
6. Recheck CMS distal to injury site

B. ELBOW
1. Check CMS distal to injury site
2. Stabilize manually proximal and distal to injury site
3. Immobilize elbow joint, upper arm and forearm with rigid splint
4. Secure in place
5. Recheck CMS distal to injury site

C. FOREARM (Radius and Ulna)
1. Check CMS distal to injury site
2. Stabilize manually proximal and distal to injury site
3. Place a rigid splint on the entire anterior aspect of the forearm to maintain alignment and secure in place
4. Wrap splint and forearm with bandage leaving finger tips exposed
5. Apply sling and swathe to keep elbow immobilized and hand pointing slightly upward toward opposite shoulder
6. Recheck CMS distal to injury site

D. WRIST
1. Check CMS distal to injury site
2. Stabilize manually proximal and distal to injury site
3. Immobilize wrist with hand in position of function
4. Secure splint and forearm with bandage leaving wrist and finger tips exposed
5. Recheck CMS distal to injury site

E. HAND
1. Check CMS distal to injury site
2. Stabilize manually proximal and distal to injury site
3. Immobilize hand in position of function
4. Place a rigid splint on the entire anterior aspect of the forearm to maintain alignment and secure in place, leaving finger tips exposed
5. Keep hand elevated
6. Recheck CMS distal to injury site

POINTS OF EMPHASIS: (Lower Extremities)
- Apply and maintain manual stabilization of the extremity until the splinting process is complete
- Align severely angulated fractures with gentle traction unless resistance is felt
- Do not attempt to replace protruding bone ends into the wound, if present
- Injuries involving joints should be immobilized in the position found
- Make one attempt to restore circulation distal to an injury site
- Avoid applying pressure to the injury site, whenever possible
- Watch for the development of hypovolemic shock due to internal hemorrhage associated with pelvic, hip and femur fractures
- PASG may be used as a splinting device as well as an anti-shock device per local protocol.
- Place PASG on long spinal immobilization device before positioning patient
- Do not log roll patient when moving to a rigid support device

F. PELVIC INJURIES
1. Check CMS in both lower extremities

2. Immobilize legs by tying knees and ankles together with bandages, padding between thighs and knees, unless this increases patient's pain
3. Lift and/or slide the patient as a unit on to a long spinal immobilization device or use orthopedic stretcher. DO NOT log roll patient
4. Flex the patient's knees with pillows underneath for comfort, if possible, and secure patient to long spineboard or orthopedic stretcher
5. Recheck CMS in both lower extremities

G. HIP INJURIES
1. Check CMS in both lower extremities
2. Lift and/or slide the patient as a unit onto a long spinal immobilization device or use an orthopedic stretcher. DO NOT log roll patient
3. Support the extremity in the position found using blankets, pillows or similar materials.
4. Secure the patient to the long spinal immobilization device
5. Recheck CMS in both lower extremities

H. THIGH INJURIES (Femur) TRACTION SPLINT (Hare style)
First MEDIC:
1. Take position at injured extremity out of the way of person applying splint
2. Check CMS distal to injury site
3. The ankle hitch may be applied at this time
4. Grasp and support the calf with one hand. With the other hand, grasp ankle, or ankle hitch strap, in preparation for lifting
5. Apply traction sufficient to stabilize the injured thigh until traction can be assumed by splint

Second MEDIC:
1. Adjust the length of the splint by measuring against the length of the uninjured leg and lock securely in place
2. Position leg support straps on splint with two proximal to the knee, one distal to the knee and one just proximal to the ankle hitch
3. Release traction mechanism and extend traction strap
4. Position splint under injured extremity
5. Extend or attach heel stand to support splint
6. Verify the ischial pad is firmly against the ischial tuberosity
7. Firmly secure groin strap using care not to pinch the external genitalia
8. If not previously done, apply ankle hitch to patient's ankle so as to maintain foot at right angle to leg when traction is applied
9. Attach traction mechanism to ankle hitch
10. Tighten traction mechanism until:
    a. First MEDIC reports mechanical traction equals manual traction
    b. Patient acknowledges pain relief
11. Readjust leg support straps if necessary with two proximal to the knee, one distal to the knee and one proximal to the ankle hitch
12. Secure leg support straps
13. Recheck CMS distal to injury site
14. Secure patient and splint to long spinal immobilization device

TRACTION SPLINT (Sager style)
1. Check CMS distal to injury site
2. Adjust length of splint

3. Slide groin strap under injured leg. NOTE: Splint may be applied to either the lateral or medial aspect of the leg
4. Secure the groin strap using sufficient padding to insure patient comfort
5. Estimate the size of the ankle and fold down the number of pads needed
6. Apply the ankle harness snugly around the patient's ankle
7. Extend the inner shaft of the splint by holding the shaft lock in the open position and pulling the inner shaft out until the desired amount of traction, per manufacturer's recommendations, is noted on the calibrated wheel
8. Apply the longest strap as high up on the thigh as possible
9. Apply the second longest strap as low as possible on the thigh
10. Apply the shortest strap over the ankle harness and lower leg
11. Apply figure eight strap around both ankles by slipping the strap under the ankles. Cross strap over the heel and secure buckle snugly
12. Recheck CMS distal to injury site

TRACTION SPLINT (Kendrick Traction Device)
1. Check CMS distal to injury site
2. Apply ankle hitch tightly around the leg, slightly above the ankle
3. Tighten stirrup by pulling the green tabbed strap, until snug under patient's heel
4. Apply upper thigh system by sliding the pronged portion of buckle under the leg, at the knee, and seesaw upward until positioned in groin area. Secure buckle
5. Cinch the groin strap until traction pole receptacle is positioned in line with the iliac crest
6. Extend the traction pole
7. Place traction pole along the lateral aspect of the injured leg, extending approximately eight (8) inches (one pole section) beyond the bottom of the foot
8. Insert pole end(s) into traction pole receptacle
9. Secure yellow elastic strap around knee
10. Place yellow tab end of blue cinch strap (located on ankle hitch) over the dart end of traction pole
11. Apply traction by pulling the red tab end of cinch strap until patient comfort improves
12. Apply upper (red) elastic strap and lower (green) elastic strap around patient's leg and traction pole
13. Recheck CMS distal to injury site

I. KNEE INJURIES
1. Check CMS distal to injury site
2. Splint the knee in the position found
3. Immobilize knee joint with rigid splints
4. Recheck CMS distal to injury site

J. LEG INJURIES (Tibia and/or Fibula)
1. Check CMS distal to injury site
2. Stabilize manually proximal and distal to the injury site.
3. Immobilize with rigid splint(s)
4. Secure in place
5. Recheck CMS distal to injury site

NOTE: When using board splints, apply one medial and one lateral to the leg. If using one board splint, apply to the posterior aspect of the leg.

K. ANKLE AND FOOT INJURIES
1. Check CMS distal to injury site
2. Stabilize manually proximal and distal to injury site
3. Immobilize with pillow, blanket, or appropriate commercial splinting device, leaving toes exposed
4. Elevate foot and ankle to reduce edema
5. Recheck CMS proximal and distal to injury site.

SECTION 10 – SPINAL INJURIES

DEFINITIONS:
- *Spinal Stabilization:* Keeping the head, neck, and spine inline, or limiting motion if the spine cannot be brought in line. This usually can be accomplished with the use of a well-fitting cervical collar, blanket horse collar, or rolled towel when a commercial cervical collar cannot be properly fitted. Additional equipment that can assist in spinal stabilization includes head blocks, blanket rolls, or tape. Please note that long spine boards, short spine boards, KED (or other extrication devices) and scoop stretchers are not a required component to spinal stabilization. These devices can be used for patient movement but should be removed as soon as the patient has reached the ambulance cot (if life-sustaining treatment doesn't preclude patient movement). The mattress on an ambulance cot contours to a patient's spine and provides better stabilization than a firm board while at the same time decreases pain and pressure points. Also note that if a patient is placed with the pelvis at the hinge point of the ambulance cot, the spine can remain inline while the head of the cot can be raised 15 to 30 degrees. This slight elevation can improve ventilation, improve brain perfusion, and decrease risk of aspiration.
- *Neck Pain:* Neck pain includes any stiffness or tenderness upon palpation at the posterior midline or paraspinal area of the cervical spine or back.
- *Decisional Patient:* The patient must be calm, cooperative, sober, oriented and alert. There can be no communication barriers including, but not limited to: age, language, closed head injury, deafness, intoxication, or other injury that interferes with the patient's ability to concentrate on or cooperate with the examination.

OBJECTIVES:
- To provide protection of the spinal column in a patient with suspected spinal fracture/dislocation and/or potential for spinal cord injury from blunt trauma.
- To provide spinal stabilization while maintaining a patent airway.
- To restore and maintain normal anatomical alignment of the spinal column and head.
- To provide spinal stabilization throughout all patient handling, packaging, and transport procedures.

POINTS OF EMPHASIS:
- Patients with penetrating traumatic injuries should undergo spinal stabilization if a focal neurologic deficit is noted on physical examination (Although there is little evidence of benefit, even in these cases. Follow local protocol).
- Assess circulation, movement, and sensation (CMS) prior to and following patient movement and stabilization to cot or mechanical device.
- Document patient's neurologic condition (CMS) before and after splinting or movement.
- One rescuer is responsible for stabilization of the head, neck and maintenance of the airway.
- Rescuer maintaining manual stabilization directs patient movement.
- Restoring spinal alignment may be appropriate during the spinal stabilization and immobilization process. However, if resistance to movement of the neck or spine is felt, or the patient experiences an increase in pain, stabilize the patient in the position found.
- In general, a cervical collar should be used during the stabilization/immobilization process. A cervical collar alone is not adequate for protecting the cervical spine.
- Depending on the style of the cervical color in use, the chinstrap may be more appropriately placed on the C-collar below the chin.
- When using tape to secure the patient's head to cot or long board, avoid applying sticky side of tape to eyebrows.

- If spinal stabilization has been completed with a mechanical device, the device may be positioned to assist in maintaining a patent airway.
- Patients may be immobilized to a long or short immobilization device using straps, tape, cravats, Velcro closures, commercial devices, etc. Appropriate padding such as blankets, towels, dressings, etc., may be needed to prevent movement of the patient in or on the immobilization device.
- Consider padding board for patient comfort.
- Decisional patients have the right to refuse aspects of treatment, including spinal stabilization. If the patient refuses spinal stabilization, after being informed of the possible permanent paralysis, document the patient's refusal in your medical record.

SKILLS:

A. SPINAL STABILIZATION ASSESSMENT FOR EXCLUSION OR INCLUSION
   1. A complete patient assessment will be completed on all trauma patients including those who are potential candidates for spinal stabilization exclusion under this section.
   2. This section does not exclude any patient from spinal stabilization if the EMS personnel feels spinal stabilization precautions are warranted.
   3. Documentation on the patient care report should reflect positive and negative physical findings as outlined below:
   4. Spinal stabilization may be excluded if the patient meets **ALL** of the following criteria and is allowed by local protocol:
      a. The traumatic incident is minor with no significant mechanism of injury, vehicle or environmental damage.
      b. There are no high risk mechanism trauma criteria present from the universal trauma field triage guidelines.
      c. The patient does not have significant head or facial trauma.
      d. The decisional patient denies neck or spine pain or tenderness with or without palpation.
      e. There is no history of loss of consciousness or altered mental status associated with the trauma.
      f. There is no history of new or temporary neurologic deficit such as numbness or weakness in an extremity.
      g. The patient does not appear to be under the influence of drugs or alcohol.
      h. There are no significant distracting injuries that may distract the patient from perceiving pain or tenderness. NOTE: Distracting injuries include, but are not limited to, fractures, lacerations, burns, crush injuries, and other causes of severe or distracting pain.
   5. If the patient has met all of the above criteria, have the patient rotate their head 45 degrees to both sides. If there still is no discomfort, spinal stabilization is not required.

B. SPINAL STABILIZATION – AMBULATORY PATIENT, STANDING
   1. Check CMS in all four extremities.
   2. Patient may ambulate to ambulance cot and lie down, with pelvis near the hinge point of the cot.
   3. Place an appropriate sized cervical collar on the patient.
   4. Instruct the patient to hold their head still. Secure the head to the cot mattress with tape across the forehead if the patient is not following commands to keep head still.
   5. Elevate the head of cot 15-30 degrees if possible for comfort.
   6. Re-check CMS in all four extremities.

C. SPINAL STABILIZATION – AMBULATORY PATIENT, SITTING
1. Check CMS in all four extremities.
2. Allow patient to self-extricate / stand with assistance as needed.
3. Patient may ambulate to ambulance cot and lie down, with pelvis near the hinge point of the cot.
4. Instruct the patient to hold their head still. Secure the head to the cot mattress with tape across the forehead if the patient is not following commands to keep head still.
5. Elevate the head of cot 15-30 degrees if possible for comfort.
6. Re-check CMS in all four extremities.

D. SPINAL STABILIZATION – NON-AMBULATORY PATIENT, SITTING
1. First Medic:
   a. Stabilize and support the head in a neutral position.
   b. Maintain stabilization until patient's head is secured with tape.
2. Second and third Medic:
   a. Check CMS in all four extremities.
   b. Place an appropriate sized cervical collar on the patient.
   c. Rotate the patient as a unit, maintaining spinal alignment and manual stabilization.
   d. Lay patient onto board and slide patient to the top of the long board. A KED or other device should only be used if a vertical rescue is needed and the patient has to be lifted in a seated fashion when horizontal entry is not possible.
   e. Temporarily secure the patient to the long board when carrying the patient.
   f. Temporarily secure the patient's forehead to the board with tape and release manual stabilization.
   g. Restrain patient's extremities in appropriate manner, if needed for safety.

3. To transfer patient from long board to the ambulance cot:
   a. Position cot level at Medic's waist height.
   b. Place long board (with patient) on the foot of the cot; long board should be half on cot.
   c. Medic supports foot end of long board.
   d. Medics two and three
      1) Unstrap patient from long board, including removing forehead tape.
      2) Stand on opposite sides of the cot / patient, facing the head of the cot and grasp the patient under the axilla with their arm closest to the cot.
      3) Place the palm of the hand, which is furthest away from the patient, on the patient's ear to maintain manual cervical stabilization. A 4th Medic, if available, could take manual stabilization from the head of the cot.
      4) Place their cot side foot near wheel of the cot to stabilize it. 4th Medic can assist in holding the cot in place while holding manual stabilization from the head of the cot.
      5) Slide the patient from the long board onto the cot while 1st Medic continues to hold the foot of the long board in place.
   e. It is important to be sure that the patient is slid up far enough on the cot such that the patient's pelvis is near the hinge point of the cot. This can allow for elevation of the patient's head without bending the lumbar spine.
   f. Instruct the patient to hold head still. Secure head to cot mattress with tape across the forehead if the patient is not following commands to keep their head still.
   g. The patient's head may be elevated 15-30 degrees to improve ability to breath and decrease intracranial pressure.
   h. Secure the patient to the cot with 4 straps.
4. Re-check CMS in all four extremities

E. LOG ROLL TO LONG BOARD – NON-AMBULATORY PATIENT, SUPINE (3 MEDICS REQUIRED)

POINT OF EMPHASIS:
- Scoop stretcher has less spinal movement than log rolling for the supine patient.

SKILL:
1. First Medic:
   a. Stabilize and support the head in a neutral position.
   b. Maintain stabilization until patient's head is secured with tape.
2. Second and third Medic:
   a. Check CMS in all four extremities.
   b. Place an appropriate sized cervical collar on the patient.
   c. Tie patient's lower extremities together
   d. Second rescuer raises patient's near arm over patient's head to prevent arm from obstructing roll or places arm along patient's side with hand against thigh
   e. Second and third rescuer s reach across patient and place their hands along patient's body evenly spaced between shoulder and knees
   f. On signal from first rescuer, second and third rescuer s roll patient toward them, maintaining spinal alignment
   g. Second and third rescuers each use hand closest to patient's feet to position the long immobilization device on the floor next to the patient's back
   h. On signal from first rescuer, all roll the patient back onto long immobilization device and lower arm to side
   i. If centering of the patient is necessary; on signal from first rescuer, slide patient with gentle even motion while maintaining spinal alignment
   j. Third rescuer secures patient to long immobilization device at chest, pelvis, thighs, and below knees, padding as necessary
   k. Second rescuer secures patient's head to long immobilization device, padding as necessary to maintain neutral alignment
   l. First rescuer may then release manual stabilization
   m. Recheck CMS in all four extremities

F. LOG ROLL TO LONG BOARD – NON-AMBULATORY PATIENT, PRONE (3 MEDICS REQUIRED)

SKILL:
1. First Medic:
   a. Stabilize and support the head in a neutral position.
   b. Maintain stabilization until patient's head is secured with tape.
2. Second and third Medic:
   a. Check CMS in all four extremities.
   b. Tie patient's lower extremities together
   c. Place long spinal immobilization device parallel to the patient so the back of the patient's head is next to the board
   d. Both rescuers kneel on board facing the patient with second rescuer at the patient's chest and third rescuer at the patient's thighs
   e. Second rescuer raises patient's arm nearest the device and positions it over the patient's head or alongside the patient's body with the hand against the thigh
   f. Second and third rescuer s reach across patient and place their hands along patient's body evenly spaced between shoulder and knees

- g. On signal from first rescuer, second and third rescuer s roll patient toward them onto long immobilization device
- h. As patient is rolled, first rescuer brings head into neutral position, if possible, achieving spinal alignment (If resistance is felt, head is stabilized at that point)
- i. If centering of the patient is necessary; on signal from first rescuer, slide patient with gentle even motion while maintaining spinal alignment
- j. Third rescuer secures patient to long immobilization device at chest, pelvis, thighs, and below knees, padding as necessary
- k. Second rescuer selects and applies an appropriately-sized cervical collar, then secures patient's head to long immobilization device, padding as necessary to maintain neutral alignment
- l. First rescuer may then release manual stabilization
- m. Recheck CMS in all four extremities

G. MOVEMENT OF A SUPINE PATIENT TO A COT USING A SCOOP STRETCHER
1. Check CMS in all four extremities
2. Select and apply cervical collar
3. Adjust stretcher to height of patient
4. Place one half of stretcher on each side of patient
5. Slide stretcher halves under patient and latch head end together
6. Close foot end of stretcher being careful not to pinch patient
7. Temporarily secure the patient to scoop stretcher for moving patient.
8. Temporarily secure the patient's forehead
9. Position the scoop stretcher so the paint's pelvis is near the hinge point of the cot. This can allow for elevation of the patient's head without bending the lumbar spine.
10. Open the foot end of the stretcher.
11. Open the head end of the stretcher.
12. Remove the 2 halves without disturbing spinal alignment.
13. Instruct the patient to hold their head still. Secure the head to the cot mattress with tape across the forehead if the patient is not following commands to keep head still.
14. Elevate the head of cot 15-30 degrees if possible for comfort.
15. Secure patient to cot.
16. Re-check CMS in all four extremities.

H. KENDRICK EXTRICATION DEVICE (KED)

POINTS OF EMPHASIS:
- A KED or other commercial extrication device should only be use for a seated patient that requires vertical extrication.
- Groin straps may be utilized in the "crisscross" or "same side" configuration.

SKILLS:
1. First rescuer:
   a. Stabilize and support the head in a neutral position
   b. Maintain stabilization until patient's head is secured to KED
2. Second rescuer:
   a. Check CMS in all four extremities
   b. Assist in repositioning the patient's body to a neutral position, as necessary
   c. Select and apply an appropriately sized cervical collar

    d. Prepare and position KED behind patient (Request additional help in positioning patient if necessary)
    e. Secure KED with center and bottom chest straps. Assure firm contact of device with lower back and armpits
    f. Pad any void between patient's head and the device to preserve neutral alignment as is necessary
    g. Secure head to device; first strap over forehead, second strap over chin

NOTE: The chin strap may be omitted or removed if airway compromise exists

    h. First MEDIC may now release manual stabilization
    i. Recheck CMS in all four extremities

3. Both rescuers
    j. Secure groin and top chest straps, if not done previously
    k. Tie hands together and lower extremities together, if necessary
    l. Position long immobilization device adjacent to patient
    m. Slide and pivot patient; support patient at thighs and with device handles
    n. Lower patient to long immobilization device; maintain legs in flexed position
    o. Move patient to head of long immobilization device
    p. Release groin straps and lower the patient's legs to the long immobilization device. Loosen top chest strap as necessary to facilitate breathing and patient comfort
    q. Secure patient to long immobilization device at chest, pelvis, thighs, and below knees, padding as necessary
    r. Recheck CMS in all four extremities

I SPINAL INJURY – XP-ONE (xp-1) (optional)

1. First rescuer
    a. Stabilize and support the head in a neutral position
    b. Maintain stabilization until patient's head is secured to XP-1

2. Second rescuer
    c. Check CMS in all four extremities
    d. Assist in repositioning the patient's body to a neutral position, as necessary
    e. Apply Med-Spec extrication collar
    f. Prepare and position XP-1 behind patient (Request additional help in positioning patient if necessary)
    g. Secure XP-1 with center and bottom chest straps. Assure firm contact of device with lower back and armpits
    h. Secure head to device, choose appropriate tabs and attach them to the Velcro on both sides of the collar. Place forehead pad on patient and attach tabs

3. Both rescuers
    i. Secure groin straps
    j. Apply top chest strap; draw shoulder straps down, loop Velcro around top on top and middle chest straps and secure in place
    k. Position long immobilization device adjacent to patient
    l. Slide and pivot patient; support patient at thighs and with device handles
    m. Lower patient to long immobilization device; maintain legs in flexed position
    n. Move patient to head of long immobilization device
    o. Release groin straps and lower the patient's legs to the long immobilization device. Loosen top chest strap as necessary to facilitate breathing and patient comfort
    p. Remove chin strap, if needed, to assure an airway

        q. Secure patient to long immobilization device at chest, pelvis, thighs, and below knees, padding as necessary
        r. Recheck CMS in all four extremities

J. SLING AND SPINEBOARD
    1. First rescuer
        a. Stabilize and support the head in a neutral position
        b. Maintain manual stabilization until patient's head is secured with tape or device.
    2. Second rescuer
        a. Check CMS in all four extremities
        b. Select and apply an appropriately-sized cervical collar
        c. Position sling across chest and under armpits of patient and tighten around body
        d. Secure patient's hands together if possible
        e. Position long spineboard at slight elevation to patient's longitudinal axis. Support at this angle while pulling patient
        f. On command, pull patient slowly onto board keeping sling close to board at all times as First rescuer guides patient's body and maintains stabilization of the head
        g. As first rescuer approaches head of board, lower board gently and move back as pull is completed
        h. Secure patient to long immobilization device at chest, pelvis, thighs, and below knees, padding as necessary
        i. Secure patient's head to long spineboard, padding as necessary
        j. First rescuer may then release manual stabilization
        k. Recheck CMS in all four extremities

K. STRADDLE LIFT (4 MEDICS MINIMUM)
    1. First Rescuer
        a. Stabilize head, neck and spine in neutral position
        b. Maintain manual stabilization until patient's head is secured with tape or device.
    2. Second, Third and Fourth Rescuers
        a. Check CMS in all four extremities
        b. Select and apply an appropriately-sized cervical collar
           Second and third rescuer s straddle patient facing first rescuer
        c. Second rescuer bends and places hands under patient's chest below the shoulders
        d. Third rescuer bends and places hands under patient's pelvis
        e. Fourth rescuer positions long spineboard lengthwise at the patient's head or feet
        f. At signal from the first rescuer, second and third rescuers lift patient just enough to allow the long spineboard to pass under the patient's body
        g. Fourth rescuer slides long spineboard under patient in one smooth, unbroken movement
        h. On signal from first rescuer, second and third rescuers lower patient on the long spineboard
        i. If centering of the patient is necessary; on signal from first rescuer, slide patient with gentle even motion while maintaining spinal alignment
        j. Third rescuer secures patient to long immobilization device at chest, pelvis, thighs, and below knees, padding as necessary
        k. Second rescuer secures patient's head to long spineboard, padding as necessary to maintain neutral alignment
        l. First rescuer may then release manual stabilization
        m. Recheck CMS in all four extremities

L. HELMET REMOVAL

POINTS OF EMPHASIS:
- The ability to maintain an airway is of ultimate importance when managing helmeted patients
- Stabilization and immobilization are the only adequate protection for suspected spinal injuries
- Consideration should be given to leaving a well-fitting helmet, which allows ready access to perform all necessary airway maneuvers, in place
- Proper immobilization of patients wearing helmets and other protective equipment often requires the patient's body or head to be padded to maintain appropriate neutral position
- Glasses, microphones, head-sets or other obstructions must be removed before attempting to remove the helmet.
- If the patient is wearing other protective equipment, once the helmet is removed, care must be taken to pad between the occiput and the immobilization device to maintain the head in a neutral alignment
- Depending on the style of helmet being worn, it may be necessary to use a closed face helmet procedure to remove the helmet
- Coaching or trainer staff may be able to assist with equipment removal.
- If the patient is wearing other protective equipment, extreme care must be taken to insure spinal alignment is maintained both during the log roll and once the helmet is removed.

SKILLS:
1. Open faced helmets/half helmets
    a. From the cephalic position, first MEDIC provides manual stabilization by placing one hand on each side of the helmet with the fingers on the mandible
    b. Second MEDIC removes the face shield, then and unfastens the restraining strap
    c. Second MEDIC places one hand on each side of the patient's neck with thumbs resting against the angle of the jaw and the fingers extending behind the occiput to support the patient's head and maintain manual stabilization
    d. First MEDIC then removes the helmet by grasping the straps or edges of the helmet to spread it as it is gently pulled along the long axis of the body and tilted slightly forward
    e. Throughout the removal process, the second MEDIC maintains manual stabilization of the patient's head and neck
    f. First MEDIC resumes control of manual stabilization
    g. The second MEDIC selects and applies an appropriately-sized cervical collar in preparation for moving the patient to a long immobilization device
    h. MEDICs move patient to long immobilization device using appropriate technique as previously described in this section

2. Closed face (full face) helmet - (Minimum of three rescuers) Assumes a well fitted helmet and no immediate life-threat due to airway obstruction or respiratory arrest
    a. Patient is positioned on long spineboard using appropriate technique as described previously in this section
    b. While maintaining manual stabilization, the head end of the long immobilization device is elevated approximately three inches from the horizontal and firmly blocked in that position
    c. While the First MEDIC maintains manual stabilization from the cephalic position, the Second and Third MEDICs straddle the patient and the long spineboard
    d. Second MEDIC grasps the patient under the armpits while Third MEDIC grasps patient at the pelvis

e. On signal from the First MEDIC, the patient is moved up the long spineboard until the lower rim of the helmet is just beyond the top edge of the board
f. While the Third MEDIC continues to stabilize the patient's body, the Second MEDIC places one hand on each side of the patient's neck with thumbs resting against the angle of the jaw and the fingers extending behind the occiput to support the patient's head and maintain manual stabilization
g. Second MEDIC assumes manual stabilization of patient's head and cervical spine
h. When advised by Second MEDIC that s/he has assumed manual stabilization, First MEDIC slowly releases manual stabilization
i. First MEDIC insures that any objects which could obstruct helmet removal (glasses, microphones, headset, etc.) have been removed from the patient and/or helmet, then loosens and unfastens the helmet restraining strap
j. First MEDIC then removes the helmet by grasping the straps or edges of the helmet to spread it as it is gently pulled along the long axis of the body and tilted slightly rearward to clear the patient's nose
k. Once the lower edge of the helmet has cleared the patient's nose, the helmet is tilted slightly forward and removed
l. First MEDIC resumes manual stabilization of the patient's head and cervical spine
m. Second MEDIC grasps patient under armpits
n. On signal from First MEDIC, all MEDICs slide the patient down the long spineboard until s/he is properly positioned
o. C-collar is applied and patient is secured to long spineboard using appropriate technique as previously described in this section

3. Football Helmet (Patient supine)
    a. First MEDIC provides manual stabilization by placing one hand on each side of the helmet with the fingers on the mandible
    b. Second MEDIC removes the face shield by using paramedic shears to cut the nylon straps holding the shield in position
    c. Second MEDIC then unfastens chin strap(s) at the side snaps, removing it completely
    d. Using the closed trauma shears as a lever, the second MEDIC pries the lower lateral interior pads from the helmet and removes them
    e. If the helmet is equipped with an air bladder, the second MEDIC releases the air valve of the helmet and deflates the bladder
    f. Second MEDIC places one hand on each side of the patient's neck with the thumbs resting against the angle of the jaw and the fingers extending behind the occiput to support the patient's head and maintain neutral alignment
    g. First MEDIC then removes the helmet by grasping its edges to spread it as it is gently pulled along the long axis of the body and tilted slightly forward
    h. Throughout the removal process the second MEDIC maintains manual stabilization of the patient's head and neck
    i. First MEDIC resumes control of manual stabilization
    j. Second MEDIC selects and applies an appropriately sized cervical collar in preparation for moving the patient to a long immobilization device
    k. MEDICs move the patient to a long immobilization device using appropriate technique as previously described in this section
    l. The second MEDIC pads as necessary under the patient's head to maintain neutral alignment m. Patient is secured to long immobilization device using appropriate technique as previously described in this section

SECTION 11 – OTHER ADVANCED LIFE SUPPORT SKILLS

I. NASOGASTRIC / OROGASTRIC TUBE INSERTION

OBJECTIVES:
- To provide a means for mediation administration.
- To provide a means for gastric lavage and / decompression.
- To allow for removal of large particulate pills in cases of overdose.
- To decompress the stomach and reduce the chance of regurgitation and aspiration.
- To follow freer downward movement of the diaphragm, making ventilation easier.

POINTS OF EMPHASIS:
- Utilize general patient support care.
- For patients with suspected facial or basilar skull fracture, the tube should be inserted orally rather than nasally.

SKILLS:
A. If possible, sit patient upright for optimal neck / stomach alignment
B. Approximate the length of the nasogastric tube need by measuring from the tip of the nose to earlobe, then point halfway between the end of the sternum and navel.
C. Mark measured length with a maker or not the distance.
D. Lubricate the distal 2-4 inches (5-10 cm) of the tube with a water-soluble lubricant.
E. Insert gastric tube (Have the patient swallow to assist in insertion.
   1. For nasal insertion:
      a. Examine nostrils for deformities or obstruction to determine best side for insertion.
      b. For patient with an ETT in place, insert the nasogastric tube into the patient's nostril, directing the advancement straight back along the floor of the nasal passage.
   2. For oral insertion, insert the gastric tube into the patient's mouth, directing for advancement posteriorly.
F. Advance the tube until:
   1. The measured / marked length of the tube has been reached.
   2. Gastric contents appear in the tube.
   3. Gastric distention is relieved.
G. Check the posterior pharynx to be sure the tube is not curled up in back of the mouth.
   1. If found curled in the pharynx, withdraw and reinsert the tube, advancing it if necessary with McGill forceps under visualization with a laryngoscope and blade.
   2. Withdraw tube immediately if changes occur in patient's respiratory status.
H. Once insertion is complete, inject approximately 20-30 ml of air into the tube while listening over the stomach with a stethoscope to confirm placement.
I. Secure the tube with tape or commercial securing device.
J. If placed for suctioning stomach contents:
   1. Remove syringe from free end of tube
   2. Connect to suction
   3. Set suction pressure per local protocols.

II. THORACENTESIS

OBJECTIVES:
- To provide an open pathway into the pleural space to decompress a suspected tension pneumothorax.
- To release trapped air causing a tension pneumothorax.

POINTS OF EMPHASIS:
- Administer 100% oxygen, and ventilate the patient if necessary.
- Assess the patient to confirm the presence of a tension pneumothorax.
- Gather equipment before starting the procedure and maintain sterility of equipment. Equipment may be a kit and / or include:
    - 10 - 14 gauge 3 1/4 inch catheter
    - Antimicrobial solution for cleaning the site
    - Tape
    - 10 ml syringe
    - Heimlich valve
    - Stethoscope
    - Sharps container
    - Sterile gloves
- Complete the patient assessment to determine / confirm presence and side of the tension pneumothorax.
- To minimize risk of infection, prep the area of puncture and maintain sterility of equipment.
- If tension pneumothorax recurs (as noted by return of respiratory distress), repeat the needle decompression on the injured side.
- Document procedure and results, including any unusual circumstances and / or difficulties encountered

SKILLS:
A. Administer 100% oxygen, and ventilate the patient as needed.
B. Explain the procedure to the patient and family / friends, if appropriate.
C. Determine which side of the chest has a tension pneumothorax.
D. Locate landmarks: 2nd intercostal space between the 2nd and 3rd ribs at the mid-clavicular line.
E. Prep the area with antimicrobial solution.
F. Don sterile gloves
G. Remove the protective sheath from the catheter and confirm catheter is in place.
    1. If using a 10 ml syringe, attach it to the catheter prior to entering the skin.
    2. If using catheter only, remove the plastic cap from the needle hub.
H. Use the non-dominant hand, with sterile glove on, to re-identify the landmarks.
I. Insert the over-the-needle catheter at a 90 de4gree angle to the chest wall just above the cephalad border of the 3rd rib, advancing into the pleural space.
J. Advance the needle until you feel a "pop" while listening for a rush of air that may be released.
K. Remove the needle leaving the catheter in place.
L. Apply the Heimlich valve to the catheter hub.
M. Secure the catheter in place, taking care not crimp it.
N. Dispose of contaminated equipment appropriately.
O. Auscultate for increased breath sounds and observe for decreased respiratory distress.
P. Continually reassess the patient for desired / undesired effects.

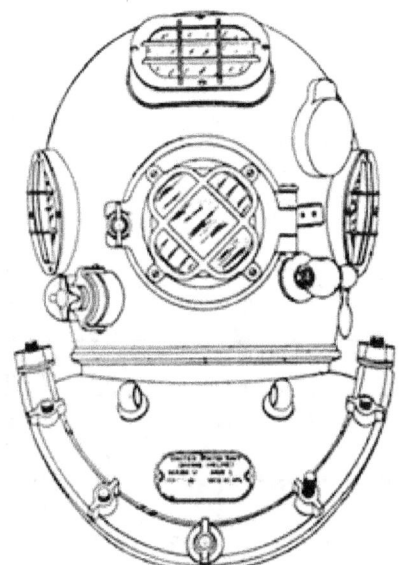

Hyperbaric Training Associates

Diver Medic

Practical Examination Skills Sheets

And

Practice Written Examination

www.divermedicaltechnician.com

MOUTH-TO-MASK WITH SUPPLEMENTAL OXYGEN

Takes or verbalizes body substance isolation precautions	1	
Connects one-way valve to mask	1	
Opens airway (manually or with adjunct)	1	
Establishes and maintains a proper mask to face seal	1	
Ventilates the patient at the proper volume and rate *(800-1200 ml per breath/10-20 breaths per minute)*	1	
Connects mask to high concentration oxygen	1	
Adjusts flow rate to greater than 15 L/min or greater	1	
Continues ventilation at proper volume and rate *(800-1200 ml per breath/10-20 breaths per minute)*	1	
NOTE: the examiner must witness ventilations for at least 30 seconds		
TOTAL:	8	

CRITICAL CRITERIA

Did not take or verbalize body substance isolation precautions

Did not adjust liter flow to 15 L/min or greater

Did not provide proper volume per breath
 (more than 2 ventilations per minute are below 800 ml)

Did not ventilate the patient at 10-20 breaths per minute

Did not allow for complete exhalation

AIRWAY MAINTENANCE
OROPHARYNGEAL AIRWAY

Takes or verbalizes body substance isolation precautions	1	
Selects appropriate size airway	1	
Measures airway	1	
Inserts airway without pushing the tongue posteriorly	1	
NOTE: The examiner must advise the candidate that the patient is gagging and becoming conscious		
Removes oropharyngeal airway	1	

SUCTION

NOTE: The examiner must advise the candidate to suction the patient's oropharynx/nasopharynx		
Turns on/prepares suction device	1	
Assures presence of mechanical suction	1	
Inserts suction tip without suction	1	
Applies suction to the oropharynx/nasopharynx	1	

NASOPHARYNGEAL AIRWAY

NOTE: The examiner must advise the candidate to insert a nasopharyngeal airway		
Selects appropriate size airway	1	
Measures airway	1	
Verbalizes lubrication of the nasal airway	1	
Fully inserts the airway with the bevel facing toward the septum	1	
TOTAL:	13	

CRITICAL CRITERIA

Did not take or verbalize body substance isolation precautions
Did not obtain a patent airway with the oropharyngeal airway
Did not obtain a patent airway with the nasopharyngeal airway

OXYGEN ADMINISTRATION

Takes or verbalizes body substance isolation precautions	1	
Assembles regulator to tank	1	
Opens tank	1	
Checks for leaks	1	
Checks tank pressure	1	
Attaches nonrebreather mask	1	
Prefills reservoir	1	
Adjusts liter flow to 15 L/min or greater	1	
Applies and adjusts mask to the patient's face	1	
NOTE: The examiner must advise the candidate to apply a nasal cannula to the patient.		
Attaches nasal cannula to oxygen	1	
Adjusts liter flow up to 6 L/min	1	
Applies nasal cannula to the patient	1	
NOTE: The examiner must advise the candidate to discontinue oxygen therapy.		
Removes the nasal cannula	1	
Shuts off the regulator	1	
Relieves the pressure within the regulator	1	
TOTAL:	15	

CRITICAL CRITERIA

    Did not take or verbalize body substance isolation precautions
    Did not assemble the tank and regulator without leaks
    Did not adjust the device to the correct liter flow for the non-rebreather mask (15 L/min)
    Did not prefill the reservoir bag
    Did not adjust the device to the correct liter flow for the nasal cannula (up to 6 L/min)

Cardiac Arrest Management/AED

ASSESSMENT		
Takes or verbalizes body substance isolation precautions	1	
Briefly questions rescuer about arrest events	1	
Directs rescuer to stop CPR	1	
Verifies absence of spontaneous pulse	1	
Turns on defibrillator power	1	
Attaches automated defibrillator to patient	1	
Ensures all individuals are standing clear of the patient	1	
Initiates analysis of rhythm	1	
Delivers shock (up to three successive shocks)	1	
Verifies absence of spontaneous pulse	1	
TRANSITION		
Directs resumption of CPR	1	
Gathers additional information on arrest event	1	
Confirms effectiveness of CPR (ventilation and compressions)	1	
INTEGRATION		
Directs insertion of a simple airway adjunct (oropharyngeal/nasopharyngeal)	1	
Directs ventilation of patient	1	
Assures high concentration of oxygen connected to the ventilatory adjunct.	1	
Assures CPR continues without unnecessary/prolonged interruption.	1	
Re-evaluates patient/CPR in approximately one minute	1	
Repeats defibrillator sequence	1	
TRANSPORTATION		
Verbalizes transportation of patient	1	
TOTAL:	20	

CRITICAL CRITERIA

Did not take or verbalize body substance isolation precautions
Did not evaluate the need for immediate use of the AED
Did not direct initiation/resumption of ventilation/compressions at appropriate times.
Did not assure all individuals were clear of patient before delivering each shock
Did not operate the AED properly (inability to deliver shock)

PATIENT ASSESSMENT/MANAGEMENT - MEDICAL

Takes or verbalizes body substance isolation precautions	1	
SCENE SIZE-UP		
Determines the scene is safe	1	
Determines the mechanism of injury/nature of illness	1	
Determines the number of patients	1	
Requests additional help if necessary	1	
Considers stabilization of spine	1	
INITIAL ASSESSMENT		
Verbalizes general impression of the patient	1	
Determines chief complaint/apparent life threats	1	
Determines responsiveness/level of consciousness	1	
Assesses airway and breathing	Assessment	1	
	Initiates appropriate oxygen therapy	1	
	Assures adequate ventilation	1	
Assesses circulation	Assesses/controls major bleeding	1
	Assesses pulse	1
	Assesses skin (color, temperature and condition)	1
Identifies priority patients/makes transport decision	1	
FOCUSED PHYSICAL EXAM AND HISTORY/RAPID ASSESSMENT		
Signs and Symptoms (Assess history of present illness)	1	

Respiratory	Cardiac	Altered Level of Consciousness	Allergic Reaction	Poisoning/ Overdose	Environmental Emergency	Obstetrics	Behavioral
*Onset? *Provokes? *Quality? *Radiates? *Severity? *Time? *Interventions?	*Onset? *Provokes? *Quality? *Radiates? *Severity? *Time? *Interventions?	*Description of the episode *Onset? *Duration? *Associated symptoms? *Evidence of trauma? *Interventions? *Seizures? *Fever?	*History of allergies? What were you exposed to? How were you exposed? Effects? Progressions *Interventions?	*Substance? *When did you Ingest/become exposed? *How much did you ingest? *Over what time period? *Interventions *Estimated weight? *Effects?	*Source? *Environment? *Duration? *Loss of consciousness? *Effects - General or local?	*Are you pregnant? *How long have you been pregnant? *Pain or contractions? *Bleeding or discharge? *Do you feel the need to push? *Last menstrual period? *Crowning?	*How do you feel? *Determine suicidal tendencies *Is the patient a threat to self or others? *Is there a medical problem? *Past medical history? *Interventions? *Medications?

Allergies	1
Medications	1
Past medical history	1
Last meal	1
Events leading to present illness (rule out trauma)	1
Performs focused physical examination Assesses affected body part/system or, if indicated, completes rapid assessment	1
VITALS (Obtains baseline vital signs)	1
INTERVENTIONS Obtains medical direction or verbalizes standing order for medication interventions and verbalizes proper additional intervention/treatment	1
TRANSPORT (Re-evaluates transport decision)	1
Completes detailed physical examination	1

ONGOING ASSESSMENT (verbalized)		
Repeats initial assessment	1	
Repeats vital signs	1	
Repeats focused assessment regarding patient complaint or injuries	1	
Checks interventions	1	
	31	

TOTAL:

CRITICAL CRITERIA

Did not take or verbalize body substance isolation precautions if necessary
Did not determine scene safety
Did not obtain medical direction or verbalize standing orders for medication interventions
Did not provide high concentration of oxygen
Did not evaluate and find conditions of airway, breathing, circulation
Did not manage/provide airway, breathing, hemorrhage control or treatment for shock
Did not differentiate patient's needing transportation versus continued assessment at the scene
Does detailed or focused history/physical examination before assessing airway, breathing and circulation

EPINEPHRINE AUTO-INJECTOR

Takes or verbalizes body substance isolation	1
Contacts medical direction for authorization	1
Obtains patient's auto-injector	1
Assures injector is prescribed for the patient	1
Checks medication for expiration date	1
Checks medication for cloudiness or discoloration	1
Removes safety cap from the injector	1
Selects appropriate injection site (thigh or shoulder)	1
Pushes injector firmly against site	1
Holds injector against site for a minimum of ten (10) seconds	1
Properly discards auto-injector	1
Verbalizes monitoring the patient while transporting	1
TOTAL:	12

CRITICAL CRITERIA:
Did not contact medical direction for authorization
Did not check medication for prescription, cloudiness or discoloration
Did not use an appropriate injection site
Used the injector against the injection site for ten (10) seconds or longer
Did not discard auto-injector into appropriate container

PATIENT ASSESSMENT/MANAGEMENT - TRAUMA

Takes or verbalizes body substance isolation precautions		1	
SCENE SIZE-UP			
Determines the scene is safe		1	
Determines the mechanism of injury		1	
Determines the number of patients		1	
Requests additional help if necessary		1	
Considers stabilization of spine		1	
INITIAL ASSESSMENT			
Verbalizes general impression of patient		1	
Determines chief complaint/apparent life threats		1	
Determines responsiveness		1	
Assesses airway and breathing	Initiates appropriate oxygen therapy Assures adequate ventilation Injury management	1 1 1	
Assesses circulation	Assesses for and controls major bleeding Assesses pulse Assesses skin	1 1 1	
Identifies priority patients/makes transport decision		1	
FOCUSED PHYSICAL EXAM AND HISTORY/RAPID TRAUMA ASSESSMENT			
Selects appropriate assessment (focused or rapid assessment)		1	
Obtains baseline vital signs		1	
Obtains S.A.M.P.L.E. history		1	
DETAILED PHYSICAL EXAMINATION			
Assesses the head	Inspects and palpates the scalp and ears Assesses the eyes Assesses the facial area	1 1 1	
Assesses the neck	Inspects and palpates the neck Assesses for JVD Assesses for tracheal deviation	1 1 1	
Assesses the chest	Inspects / Palpates Auscultates the chest	2 1	
Assesses the abdomen/pelvis	Assesses the abdomen Assesses the pelvis Verbalizes assessment of genitalia/perineum	1 1 1	
Assesses the extremities	1 point for each extremity includes inspection, palpation, and assessment of pulses, sensory and motor activities	4	
Assesses the posterior	Assesses thorax Assesses lumbar	1 1	
Manages secondary injuries and wounds appropriately 1 point for appropriate management of each injury/wound up to a maximum of 2 points		2	
Verbalizes reassessment of the vital signs		1	
		40	

TOTAL:

CRITICAL CRITERIA

　Did not assess for spinal protection
　Did not provide for spinal protection when indicated
　Did not provide high concentration of oxygen
　Did not evaluate and find conditions of airway, breathing, circulation (hypoperfusion)
　Did not manage/provide airway, breathing, hemorrhage control or treatment for shock (hypoperfusion)
　Did not differentiate patient's needing transportation versus continued on scene survey
　Does other detailed physical examination before assessing airway, breathing and circulation
　Did not transport patient within ten (10) minute time limit

BLEEDING CONTROL/SHOCK MANAGEMENT

Takes or verbalizes body substance isolation precautions	1	
Applies direct pressure to the wound	1	
Elevates the extremity	1	
Applies a dressing to the wound	1	
Bandages the wound	1	
Note: The examiner must now inform the candidate that the wound is still continuing to bleed.		
Applies an additional dressing to the wound	1	
Note: The examiner must now inform the candidate that the wound is still continuing to bleed. The second dressing does not control the bleeding.		
Locates and applies pressure to appropriate arterial pressure point	1	
Note: The examiner must now inform the candidate that the bleeding is controlled and the patient is in compensatory shock.		
Applies high concentration oxygen	1	
Properly positions the patient	1	
Initiates steps to prevent heat loss from the patient	1	
Indicates need for immediate transportation	1	
TOTAL:	11	

CRITICAL CRITERIA

　Did not take or verbalize body substance isolation precautions
　Did not apply high concentration of oxygen
　Applies tourniquet before attempting other methods of bleeding control
　Did not control hemorrhage in a timely manner
　Did not indicate a need for immediate transportation

IMMOBILIZATION SKILLS
LONG BONE

Takes or verbalizes body substance isolation precautions	1	
Directs application of manual stabilization	1	
Assesses motor, sensory and distal circulation	1	
NOTE: The examiner acknowledges present and normal		
Measures splint	1	
Applies splint	1	
Immobilizes the joint above the injury site	1	
Immobilizes the joint below the injury site	1	
Secures the entire injured extremity	1	
Immobilizes hand/foot in the position of function	1	
Reassesses motor, sensory and distal circulation	1	
Note: The examiner acknowledges present and normal		
TOTAL:	10	

CRITICAL CRITERIA

Grossly moves injured extremity
Did not immobilize adjacent joints
Did not assess motor, sensory and distal circulation after splinting

IMMOBILIZATION SKILLS
JOINT INJURY

Takes or verbalizes body substance isolation precautions	1
Directs application of manual stabilization of the injury	1
Assesses motor, sensory and distal circulation	1
NOTE: The examiner acknowledges present and normal	
Selects proper splinting material	1
Immobilizes the site of the injury	1
Immobilizes bone above injured joint	1
Immobilizes bone below injured joint	1
Reassesses motor, sensory and distal circulation	1
NOTE: The examiner acknowledges present and normal	
TOTAL:	**8**

CRITICAL CRITERIA

Did not support the joint so that the joint did not bear distal weight

Did not immobilize bone above and below injured joint

Did not reassess motor, sensory and distal circulation after splinting

IMMOBILIZATION SKILLS
TRACTION SPLINTING

Takes or verbalizes body substance isolation precautions	1	
Directs application of manual stabilization of the injured leg	1	
Directs the application of manual traction	1	
Assesses motor, sensory and distal circulation	1	
NOTE: The examiner acknowledges present and normal.		
Prepares/adjusts splint to the proper length	1	
Positions the splint at the injured leg	1	
Applies the proximal securing device (e.g..ischial strap)	1	
Applies the distal securing device (e.g..ankle hitch)	1	
Applies mechanical traction	1	
Positions/secures the support straps	1	
Re-evaluates the proximal/distal securing devices	1	
Reassesses motor, sensory and distal circulation	1	
NOTE: The examiner acknowledges present and normal.		
NOTE: The examiner must ask candidate how he/she would prepare the patient for transportation.		
Verbalizes securing the torso to the long board to immobilize the hip	1	
Verbalizes securing the splint to the long board to prevent movement of the splint	1	
	14	

TOTAL:

CRITICAL CRITERIA

Loss of traction at any point after it is assumed
Did not reassess motor, sensory and distal circulation after splinting
The foot is excessively rotated or extended after splinting
Did not secure the ischial strap before taking traction
Final immobilization failed to support the femur or prevent rotation of the injured leg
Secures leg to splint before applying mechanical traction

SPINAL IMMOBILIZATION
LYING PATIENT

Takes or verbalizes body substance isolation precautions	1	
Directs assistant to place/maintain head in neutral in-line position	1	
Directs assistant to maintain manual immobilization of the head	1	
Assesses motor, sensory and distal circulation in extremities	1	
Applies appropriate size extrication collar	1	
Positions the immobilization device appropriately	1	
Moves patient onto device without compromising the integrity of the spine	1	
Applies padding to voids between the torso and the board as necessary	1	
Immobilizes the patient's torso to the device	1	
Evaluates and pads behind the patient's head as necessary	1	
Immobilizes the patient's head to the device	1	
Secures the patient's legs to the device	1	
Secures the patient's arms to the device	1	
Reassesses motor, sensory and distal circulation in extremities	1	
TOTAL:	14	

CRITICAL CRITERIA

Did not immediately direct or take manual immobilization of the head
Releases or orders release of manual immobilization before it was maintained mechanically
Patient manipulated or moved excessively causing potential spinal compromise
Device moves excessively up, down, left or right on patient's torso
Head immobilization allows for excessive movement
Upon completion of immobilization, head is not in the neutral position
Did not reassess motor, sensory and distal circulation after immobilization
Immobilizes head to the board before securing torso

SPINAL IMMOBILIZATION
SEATED PATIENT

Takes or verbalizes body substance isolation precautions	1	
Directs assistant to place/maintain head in neutral in-line position	1	
Directs assistant to maintain manual immobilization of the head	1	
Assesses motor, sensory and distal circulation in extremities	1	
Applies appropriate size extrication collar	1	
Positions the immobilization device behind the patient	1	
Secures the device to the patient's torso	1	
Evaluates torso fixation and adjusts as necessary	1	
Evaluates and pads behind the patient's head as necessary	1	
Secures the patient's head to the device	1	
Verbalizes moving the patient to a long board	1	
Reassesses motor, sensory and distal circulation in extremities	1	
TOTAL:	12	

CRITICAL CRITERIA
Did not immediately direct or take manual immobilization of the head
Releases or orders release of manual immobilization before it was maintained mechanically
Patient manipulated or moved excessively causing potential spinal compromise
Device moves excessively up, down, left or right on patient's torso
Head immobilization allows for excessive movement
Torso fixation inhibits chest rise resulting in respiratory compromise
Upon completion of immobilization, head is not in the neutral position
Did not reassess motor, sensory and distal circulation after immobilization
Immobilized head to the board before securing the torso

VENTILATORY MANAGEMENT
ENDOTRACHEAL INTUBATION

Takes or verbalizes body substance isolation precautions		1	
Opens airway manually		1	
Elevates tongue and inserts simple airway adjunct (oropharyngeal or nasopharyngeal airway)		1	
NOTE: The examiner now informs the candidate no gag reflex is present and the patient accepts the adjunct			
**Ventilates the patient immediately using a BVM device unattached to O2		1	
**Hyperventilates the patient with room air		1	
NOTE: The examiner now informs the candidate that ventilation is being performed without difficulty			
Attaches the oxygen reservoir to the BVM		1	
Attaches BVM to high flow oxygen		1	
Ventilates the patient at the proper volume and rate (800-1200 ml per breath/10-20 breaths per minute)		1	
NOTE: After 30 seconds, the examiner auscultates and reports breath sounds are present and equal bilaterally and medical control has ordered intubation. The examiner must now take over ventilation.			
Directs assistant to hyperventilate patient		1	
Identifies/selects proper equipment for intubation		1	
Checks equipment	Checks for cuff leaks	1	
	Checks laryngoscope operation	1	
NOTE: The examiner must remove the OPA and move out of the way when the candidate is prepared to intubate			
Positions the head properly		1	
Inserts the laryngoscope blade while displacing the tongue		1	
Elevates the mandible with the laryngoscope		1	
Introduces the ET tube and advances it to the proper depth		1	
Inflates the cuff to the proper pressure and disconnects the syringe		1	
Directs ventilation of the patient		1	
Confirms proper placement by auscultation and over the epigastrium		1	
NOTE: The examiner must ask, "If you had proper placement, what would you expect to hear?"			
Secures the ET tube (*may be verbalized*)		1	
TOTAL:		20	

CRITICAL CRITERIA
Did not take or verbalize body substance isolation precautions
Did not initiate ventilations within 30 seconds after applying gloves or interrupts ventilations for greater than 30 seconds at any time.
Did not voice or provide high oxygen concentrations (15 L/min or greater)
Did not ventilate patient at a rate of at least 10/minute
Did not provide adequate volume per breath (maximum of 2 errors/minute permissible)
Did not hyperventilate the patient prior to intubation
Did not successfully intubate within 3 attempts
Used the patients teeth as a fulcrum
Did not assure proper tube placement by auscultation bilaterally and over the epigastrium
If used, the stylet extended beyond the end of the ET tube
Inserts any adjunct in a manner that would be dangerous to the patient

VENTILATORY MANAGEMENT
DUAL LUMEN AIRWAY DEVICE (PTL OR COMBI-TUBE) INSERTION FOLLOWING AN UNSUCCESSFUL ENDOTRACHEAL INTUBATION ATTEMPT

Continues body substance isolation precautions	1	
Confirms the patient is being properly ventilated	1	
Directs assistant to hyperventilate the patient	1	
Checks/prepares airway device	1	
Lubricates distal tip of the device (*may be verbalized*)	1	
Removes the oropharyngeal airway	1	
Extends the patient's head	1	
Performs a tongue-jaw lift	1	
Inserts airway device to proper depth	1	
Inflates pharyngeal and distal cuffs	1	
Removes syringe	1	
Ventilates through proper first lumen	1	
Confirms placement by observing chest rise and auscultating over the epigastrium and bilaterally over the chest	1	
NOTE: The examiner states, "You do not see rise and fall of the chest and hear sounds only over the epigastrium."		
Ventilates through the alternate lumen	1	
Confirms placement by observing chest rise and auscultating over the epigastrium and bilaterally over the chest	1	
NOTE: The examiner confirms adequate chest rise, bilateral breath sounds and absent sounds over the epigastrium.		
Secures tube at the appropriate step in sequence	1	
TOTAL:	**16**	

CRITICAL CRITERIA
Did not take or verbalize body substance isolation precautions.
Interrupts ventilation for greater than 30 seconds.
Did not direct hyperventilation of the patient prior to placement of the device.
Did not assure proper placement of the device.
Did not successfully ventilate patient.
Did not provide high flow oxygen (15 L/min or greater)
Inserts any adjunct in a manner that would be dangerous to the patient

VENTILATORY MANAGEMENT
ESOPHAGEAL OBTURATOR AIRWAY INSERTION FOLLOWING AN UNSUCCESSFUL ENDOTRACHEAL INTUBATION ATTEMPT

Continues body substance isolation precautions	1	
Confirms the patient is being properly ventilated	1	
Directs assistant to hyperventilate the patient	1	
Identifies/selects proper equipment	1	
Assembles airway	1	
Tests cuff	1	
Inflates mask	1	
Lubricates tube (*may be verbalized*)	1	
Removes the oropharyngeal airway	1	
Positions head properly with neck in the neutral or slightly flexed position	1	
Grasps and elevates tongue and mandible	1	
Inserts tube in the same direction as the curvature of the pharynx	1	
Advances tube until the mask is sealed against the face	1	
Ventilates the patient while maintaining a tight mask seal	1	
Confirms placement by observing chest rise and auscultating over the epigastrium and bilaterally over the chest	1	
NOTE: The examiner confirms adequate chest rise, bilateral breath sounds and absent sounds over the epigastrium		
Inflates the cuff to the proper pressure and disconnects the syringe	1	
Continues ventilation of the patient	1	
Total:	**17**	

Critical Criteria
Did not take or verbalize body substance isolation precautions
Interrupts ventilation for more than 30 seconds
Did not direct hyperventilation of the patient prior to placement of the device
Did not assure proper placement of the device
Did not successfully ventilate the patient
Did not provide high flow oxygen (15 L/min or greater)
Inserts any adjunct in a manner that would be dangerous to the patient

Skills Check-Off

IM Medication (Adult)

Candidate:_____ Examiner:_____

Date:_____ Signature:_____

Time Started:_____

	Points Possible	Points Awarded
Takes, or verbalizes, body substance isolation precautions	1	
Confirms correct patient	1	
Confirms Allergies	1	
Checks selected medication: Proper medication, Concentration, Expiration Date	1	
Attaches appropriate size needle to syringe to draw up medication (If syringe is prefilled skip this step and the following step, award points automatically for the two steps)	1	
Draws up appropriate amount of medication, dispels air, and insures proper measurement of medication	1	
Reaffirms medication	1	
Attaches appropriate needle to syringe for injection	1	
Dispels air from needle (Unless performing a Z-Track)	1	
Candidate verbalizes the most common anatomical locations and associated needle sizes to administer the medication and maximum amounts that can be given at each location	1	
Candidate selects injection site, locates correct anatomical position, and cleanses with alcohol	1	
Candidate stabilizes site of injection	1	
Insert needle at a 90 degree angle	1	
Aspirates for blood	1	
Injects medication	1	
Withdraws needle and massages injection site	1	
Disposes of needle in appropriate container	1	
Verbalizes need to observe patient for desired/adverse effects of the medication	1	
Time End:_____ Total	18	

CRITICAL CRITERIA

_____ Does not immediately don or verbalize BSI
_____ Contaminates site of injection and does not take appropriate action
_____ Administers medication at inappropriate anatomical location
_____ Administers a dosage of medication greater than recommended at a anatomical location
_____ Administers improper medication (wrong medication, dosage, or concentration)

Hyperbaric Training Associates
Diver Medic Practice Section Examination

1. A patient has a blood pressure of 130/70 mm Hg. The "130" represents:
   - A) atrial contraction.
   - B) ventricular filling.
   - C) ventricular contraction.
   - D) ventricular relaxation.

2. The index of suspicion is MOST accurately defined as:
   - A) the way in which traumatic injuries occur.
   - B) a predictable pattern that leads to serious injuries.
   - C) your concern for potentially serious underlying injuries.
   - D) the detection of less obvious life-threatening injuries.

3. When a helicopter must land on a grade (uneven ground), you should:
   - A) approach the aircraft from the uphill side.
   - B) approach the aircraft from the downhill side.
   - C) attempt to approach the aircraft from behind.
   - D) move the patient to the aircraft as soon as it lands.

4. The "Chokes" is a form of _____ decompression sickness.
   - A) Pulmonary   B) Central Nervous System   C) Vestibular   D) Cerebral

5. To avoid O2 toxicity, DCS patients are given _____ to stop the O2 clock.
   - A) Water   B) Nitrous Oxide   C) Oxygen   D) Air Breaks

6. What is the therapeutic partial pressure limit for oxygen?
   - A) 1.0   B) 2.0   C) 3.0   D) 4.0

7. Frothy, pink sputum coming from a surfaced diver would indicate what?
   - A) Pulmonary Barotrauma
   - B) Moray Eel Bite
   - C) He has bitten his tongue
   - D) Sinus Squeeze

8. A fracture of the humerus just above the elbow would be described as a:
   - A) distal humerus fracture.
   - B) proximal elbow fracture.
   - C) distal forearm fracture.
   - D) proximal humerus fracture.

9. Typically, decompression sickness is caused by the release of what gas during ascent?
   A) Hydrogen   B) Nitrox   C) Carbon Dioxide   D) Inert Gas

10. The purpose of defibrillation is to:
    A) stop the chaotic, disorganized contraction of the cardiac cells.
    B) cause a rapid decrease in the heart rate of an unstable patient.
    C) improve the chance of cardiopulmonary resuscitation (CPR) being successful in resuscitation.
    D) prevent asystole from deteriorating into ventricular fibrillation.

11. If a pneumothorax continues to advance it will become a life-threatening
    A) Emphysemia   B) COPD   C) Tension Pneumothorax   D) Embolism

12. An adult at rest should have a respiratory rate that ranges between:
    A) 8 and 15 breaths/min.
    B) 10 and 18 breaths/min.
    C) 12 and 20 breaths/min.
    D) 16 and 24 breaths/min.

13. Early saturation diving research was conducted using which breathing medium?
    A) Nitrox 50/50   B) Nitrox 32/68   C) Heliox Mix   D) Trimix

14. Which of the following is the MOST rapidly acting medication administration route?
    A) sublingual (SL)
    B) intravenous (IV)
    C) subcutaneous (SC)
    D) intramuscular (IM)

15. Normal skin color, temperature, and condition should be:
    A) pink, warm, and dry.
    B) pale, cool, and moist.
    C) pink, warm, and moist.
    D) flushed, cool, and dry.

16. The purpose of the Sellick maneuver is to prevent:
    A) vomiting and aspiration.
    B) spasm of the vocal cords.
    C) collapsing of the trachea.
    D) airway blockage by the tongue.

17. Which of the following statements regarding multilumen airway devices is correct?
    A) They are contraindicated in patients who have experienced a severe spinal injury.
    B) Ventilations can be provided whether the device is in the trachea or the esophagus.
    C) Insertion of a multilumen airway device requires visualization of the upper airway.
    D) Multilumen airway device insertion does not require medical control authorization.

18. "Vestibular" DCS would be a problem with the divers' what?
    A) Vision   B) Speech   C) Breathing   D) Ears

19. Nitroglycerin is contraindicated in patients:
    A) who have taken up to two doses.
    B) who have experienced a head injury.
    C) with a history of an ischemic stroke.
    D) with a systolic blood pressure less than 120 mm Hg.

20. A generalized seizure is characterized by:
    A) severe twitching of all the body's muscles.
    B) a blank stare and brief lapse of consciousness.
    C) unconsciousness for greater than 30 minutes.
    D) a core body temperature of greater than 103°F (40°C).

21. Shallow water blackout occurs because _____ is _____ during the dive.
    A) Oxygen / Metabolized   C) Oxygen / Exhaled
    B) Nitrogen / Off gassed   D) Carbon Dioxide / Off gassed

22. A fracture is MOST accurately defined as a(n):
    A) total loss of function in a bone.   C) disruption in the midshaft of a bone.
    B) break in the continuity of the bone.   D) abnormality in the structure of a bone.

23. High humidity reduces the body's ability to lose heat through:
    A) radiation.   B) convection.   C) conduction.   D) evaporation.

24. The most superior portion of the sternum is called the:
    A) manubrium.   B) costal arch.   C) angle of Louis.   D) xiphoid process.

25. An open fracture is MOST accurately defined as a fracture in which:
    A) bone ends protrude through the skin.
    B) a large laceration overlies the fracture.
    C) a bullet shatters the underlying bone.
    D) the overlying skin is no longer intact.

26. Oxygen and carbon dioxide pass across the alveolar membrane in the lungs through a process called:
    A) osmosis.   B) breathing.   C) diffusion.   D) ventilation.

27. A diver at a depth of 99 fsw is said to be at
    A) 3 ata   B) 4 ata   C) 5 ata   D) 6 ata

28. The purpose of a saline lock is to:
    A) clamp off the IV tubing to decrease the rate at which the fluid flows.
    B) maintain an active IV site without running fluids through the vein.
    C) keep an IV line patent in patients who do not require medications.
    D) allow the delivery of large volumes of isotonic crystalloid solutions.

29. A pneumothorax left untreated would cause problems during a chamber ascent.
    A) True   B) False

30. When approaching a helicopter, whether the rotor blades are moving or not, you should:
    A) never duck under the body or the tail boom because the pilot cannot see you in these areas.
    B) remember that the main rotor blade is flexible and can dip as low as 5□ to 6□ from the ground.
    C) carefully approach the aircraft from the rear unless a crew member instructs you to do otherwise.
    D) approach the aircraft from the side because this will make it easier for you to access the aircraft doors.

31. Which of the following over-the-needle IV catheters has the largest diameter?
    A) 14-gauge   B) 16-gauge   C) 18-gauge   D) 20-gauge

32. Which of the following statements regarding standing orders is MOST correct?
    A) Standing orders have less legal authority than orders given via radio.
    B) Standing orders require you to contact medical control first.
    C) Standing orders only highlight the care that you may provide.
    D) Standing orders should be followed when physician contact is not possible.

33. Common signs and symptoms of heat exhaustion include all of the following, EXCEPT:
    A) nausea.   B) headache.   C) tachycardia.   D) hot, dry skin.

34. Which of the following physiologic actions does epinephrine produce when given for an allergic reaction?
    A) bronchodilation and vasodilation
    B) vasoconstriction and bronchodilation
    C) bronchoconstriction and vasoconstriction
    D) blocking of further histamine release

35. "Rapture of the Deep" is caused by the narcotic effect of what gas?
    A) Oxygen   B) Nitrogen   C) Helium   D) Hydrogen

36. When perfusion to the core of the body decreases:
    A) blood is shunted away from the skin.
    B) decreased cardiac contractility occurs.
    C) blood is diverted to the gastrointestinal tract.
    D) the voluntary nervous system releases hormones.

37. The FIRST rule of safe lifting is to:
    A) always lift with your palms facing down.
    B) spread your legs approximately 20□ apart.
    C) keep your back in a slightly curved position.
    D) keep your back in a straight, vertical position.

38. The five sections of the spinal column, in descending order, are the:
    A) thoracic, cervical, lumbar, coccygeal, and sacral.
    B) cervical, thoracic, lumbar, sacral, and coccygeal.
    C) coccygeal, sacral, lumbar, thoracic, and cervical.
    D) cervical, coccygeal, thoracic, sacral, and lumbar.

39. Skeletal muscle is also called:
    A) smooth muscle.
    B) autonomic muscle.
    C) voluntary muscle.
    D) involuntary muscle.

40. Most patients who die of anaphylaxis do so within the first _____ following exposure.
    A) 5 minutes   B) 30 minutes   C) 60 minutes   D) 90 minutes

41. The central nervous system (CNS) is composed of the:
    A) cerebellum and brain.
    B) brain and spinal cord.
    C) cerebrum and meninges.
    D) meninges and spinal cord.

42. Harsh, high-pitched inspiratory sounds are characteristic of:
    A) rales.   B) stridor.   C) rhonchi.   D) wheezing.

43. A partial-thickness burn involves the outer layer of skin and a portion of the:
    A) epidermis.   B) fatty layer.   C) muscle fascia.   D) dermal layer.

44. The goal of the primary assessment is to:
    A) determine if the patient's problem is medical or trauma.
    B) identify patients that require transport to a trauma center.
    C) determine the need to perform a head-to-toe assessment.
    D) identify and rapidly treat all life-threatening conditions.

45. Decompression Sickness is a function of what Gas Law?
    A) Boyles   B) Charles   C) Daltons   D) Henrys

46. The spinal cord exits the cranium through the:
    A) foramen magnum.
    B) vertebral foramen.
    C) foramen lamina.
    D) cauda equina.

47. The nasal cannula is MOST appropriately used in the prehospital setting:
    A) when the patient cannot tolerate a nonrebreathing mask.
    B) if the patient's nasopharynx is obstructed by secretions.
    C) if long-term supplemental oxygen administration is required.
    D) when the patient breathes primarily through his or her mouth.

48. Oxygen toxicity involves what system of the body?
    A) Cardiovascular   B) Cerebral   C) Musculoskeletal   D) Endocrine

49. Deoxygenated blood from the abdomen, pelvis, and lower extremities is returned to the right atrium via the:
    A) common iliac vein.
    B) coronary sinus vein.
    C) inferior vena cava.
    D) superior vena cava.

50. If a diver held his breath and surfaced after taking a breath from his scuba regulator at 99 fsw, the air in his lungs would expand
    A) 2 times   B) 3 times   C) 4 times   D) 5 times

51. The body's natural protective mechanisms against heat loss are:
    A) shivering and vasodilation.
    B) vasodilation and respiration.
    C) respiration and vasoconstriction.
    D) vasoconstriction and shivering.

52. What physician developed the first true decompression tables for heliox in the 1930s?
    A) Dr. Edgar End   B) Dr. Phil   C) Dr. Peter Bennett   D) Dr. Robert Goldmann

53. Inhalation occurs when the:
    A) diaphragm and intercostal muscles relax and cause an increase in intrathoracic pressure.
    B) diaphragm and intercostal muscles ascend and cause an increase in intrathoracic pressure.
    C) diaphragm and intercostal muscles contract and cause a decrease in intrathoracic pressure.
    D) diaphragm ascends and the intercostal muscles contract, causing a decrease in intrathoracic pressure.

54. The diastolic pressure represents the:
    A) average pressure against the arterial walls during a cardiac cycle.
    B) minimum amount of pressure that is always present in the arteries.
    C) increased arterial pressure that occurs during ventricular contraction.
    D) difference in pressure between ventricular contraction and relaxation.

55. Which of the following is NOT a characteristic of epinephrine?
    A) secreted naturally by the adrenal glands
    B) dilates passages in the lungs
    C) constricts blood vessels
    D) decreases heart rate and blood pressure

56. Definitive treatment for a tension pneumothorax in a chamber, at depth, is
    A) Intravenous Therapy
    B) Endotracheal Tube
    C) High Flow Oxygen
    D) Thoracic Needle Decompression

57. Signs and symptoms of a tension pneumothorax include
    A) Fever
    B) Headache
    C) Absent breath sounds on the affected side
    D) Increased minute volume

58. Common signs of a skull fracture include all of the following, EXCEPT:
    A) mastoid process bruising.
    B) ecchymosis around the eyes.
    C) noted deformity to the skull.
    D) superficial scalp lacerations.

59. US Navy Treatment Table 6A should be modified to us 50/50 nitrox or 50/50 Heliox.
    A) True B) False

60. Which of the following MOST accurately defines negligence?
    A) transport of a mentally incompetent patient against his or her will
    B) deviation from the standard of care that may result in further injury
    C) transferring patient care to a provider with a lower level of training
    D) providing care that is consistent with care provided by other EMTs

61. What maneuver should be used to open the airway of an unresponsive patient with suspected trauma?
    A) tongue-jaw lift
    B) jaw-thrust maneuver
    C) head tilt–chin lift
    D) head tilt–neck lift

62. The spread of HIV and hepatitis in the health care setting can usually be traced to:
    A) careless handling of sharps.
    B) a lack of proper immunizations.
    C) excessive blood splashing or splattering.
    D) a noncompliance with standard precautions.

63. The Gas Law which explains what is happening to a diver as he ascends is
    A) Henrys Law B) Daltons Law C) Charles Law D) Boyles Law

64. What is the partial pressure of 100% Oxygen at 60 fsw?
    A) 3.0 B) 0.75 C) 1.4 D) 2.8

65. Shallow and Deep water blackout is a function of which Gas Law?
    A) Boyles B) Charles C) Daltons D) Henrys

66. Signs of a pulmonary blast injury include:
    A) vomiting blood.
    B) coughing up blood.
    C) an irregular pulse.
    D) multiple rib fractures.

67. When immobilizing a patient on a long backboard, you should:
    A) have the patient exhale before fastening the torso straps.
    B) secure the torso and then center the patient on the board.
    C) follow the commands of the person at the patient's torso.
    D) ensure that you secure the torso before securing the head.

68. Movement or motion away from the body's midline is called:
    A) flexion.   B) extension.   C) adduction.   D) abduction.

69. The direct effect of bubbles in the intravascular spaces is
    A) Ischemia distal to the insult
    B) Ischemia proximal to the insult
    C) Ischemia lateral to the insult
    D) Ischemia feeling insulted

70. An unstable patient should be reassessed at least every:
    A) 5 minutes.   B) 10 minutes.   C) 15 minutes.   D) 20 minutes.

71. Functions of dressings and bandages include all of the following, EXCEPT:
    A) immobilization of the injury.
    B) prevention of contamination.
    C) protection from further injury.
    D) control of external hemorrhage.

72. An IO needle is inserted into the:
    A) bone.   B) distal humerus.   C) distal femur.   D) proximal fibula.

73. Separation of inert gas bubbles from soluble phase to gas phase may cause
    A) Cardiac Tamponade
    B) Subcutaneous Emphysema
    C) Intravascular Bubbles
    D) Acne

74. The left ventricle has the thickest walls because it:
    A) pumps blood to the lungs to be reoxygenated.
    B) uses less oxygen than other chambers of the heart.
    C) pumps blood into the aorta and systemic circulation.
    D) receives blood directly from the systemic circulation.

75. The primary prehospital treatment for most medical emergencies:
    A) typically does not require the EMT to contact medical control.
    B) focuses on definitive care because a diagnosis can usually be made.
    C) addresses the patient's symptoms more than the actual disease process.
    D) involves transport only until treatment can be performed at the hospital.

76. Any unresponsive trauma patient should be assumed to have:
    A) a history of diabetes mellitus.   C) a severe intracranial hemorrhage.
    B) an accompanying spinal injury.   D) internal bleeding in the abdomen.

77. Shunting from the right side of the heart to the left occurs via a
    A) Patent Foramen Ovale   C) Cardiac Tamponade
    B) Foramen Magnum   D) Deviated Septum

78. A diver at 1000 fsw is under how much absolute pressure per square inch?
    A) 545 psi   B) 459.7 psi   C) 445 psi   D) 44.5 psi

79. Hypothermia occurs when the core body temperature falls below:
    A) 98°F (37°C).   B) 95°F (35°C).   C) 90°F (32°C).   D) 88°F (31°C).

80. When a person is exposed to a cold environment:
    A) sweat is produced and is warmed when the vessels constrict.
    B) blood vessels dilate and divert blood to the core of the body.
    C) the skin becomes flushed secondary to peripheral vasodilation.
    D) peripheral vessels constrict and divert blood away from the skin.

81. The major predisposing factor to DCS after, of course, not following the tables is
    A) Diving everyday   B) Common cold   C) Fever   D) Dehydration

82. Ascent rates for a patient on a US Navy TT is how many feet per minute?
    A) 1 foot per minute
    B) 2 feet per minute
    C) 10 feet per minute
    D) 15 feet per minute

83. Which of the following would MOST likely result in hemorrhagic shock?
    A) severe vomiting
    B) liver laceration
    C) excessive sweating
    D) repeated diarrhea

84. Which of the following statements regarding blast injuries is correct?
    A) Solid organs such as the middle ear, lungs, and gastrointestinal tract are the most susceptible to pressure changes.
    B) Solid organs are relatively protected from shock wave injury but may be injured during the secondary or tertiary blast phase.
    C) Tertiary blast injuries are penetrating or non-penetrating injuries that result from flying debris, such as ordnance projectiles.
    D) The gastrointestinal tract is the organ system most sensitive to blast injuries and is the leading cause of death following an explosion.

85. Which of the following sounds indicates swelling of the upper airway?
    A) rales B) stridor C) rhonchi D) wheezing

86. A direct effect of DCS is mechanical pressure of the bubbles on the
    A) Base of the Cerebellum B) Nerve Roots C) Bladder D) Bones

87. A crackling sound produced by air bubbles under the skin is called:
    A) crepitus B) rhonchi. C) Korotkoff sounds. D) subcutaneous emphysema.

88. After receiving online orders from medical control to perform a patient care intervention, you should:
    A) perform the intervention as ordered.
    B) confirm the order in your own words.
    C) ask the physician to repeat the order.
    D) repeat the order to medical control word for word.

89. If a diver reaches the surface after a dive and becomes unconscious within 15 minutes, the problem should be considered
    A) Decompression Sickness
    B) Head Trauma
    C) Arterial Gas Embolism
    D) Skin Bends

90. Modern heliox diving had it's start in what city?
    A) London, England
    B) New York, New York
    C) Panama City, Florida
    D) Milwaukee, Wisconsin

91. In a healthy individual, the brain stem stimulates breathing on the basis of:
    A) increased oxygen levels.
    B) decreased oxygen levels.
    C) increased carbon dioxide levels.
    D) decreased carbon dioxide levels.

92. The actual exchange of oxygen and carbon dioxide occurs in the:
    A) bronchioles.
    B) alveolar sacs.
    C) apex of the lung.
    D) pulmonary capillaries.

93. If direct pressure with a sterile dressing fails to immediately stop severe bleeding from an extremity, you should apply:
    A) additional sterile dressings.
    B) a splint and elevate the extremity.
    C) a tourniquet proximal to the injury.
    D) digital pressure to a proximal artery.

94. Patients with full-thickness (third-degree) burns generally do not complain of pain because:
    A) blister formation protects the burn.
    B) he or she is generally not conscious.
    C) the nerve endings have been destroyed.
    D) subcutaneous vessels are usually clotted.

95. Hypoperfusion is another name for:
    A) shock.   B) cyanosis.   C) hypoxemia.   D) cellular death.

96. Endotracheal intubation is MOST accurately defined as:
    A) inserting a tube through the mouth and in between the vocal cords.
    B) inserting a tube into the trachea to maintain the airway and ventilate.
    C) inserting a suction catheter into the trachea to remove thick secretions.
    D) blindly inserting a tube through the nose and into the tracheal opening.

97. The primary purpose for splinting a musculoskeletal injury is to:
    A) prevent further injury.
    B) maximize distal circulation.
    C) make the patient comfortable.
    D) facilitate ambulance transport.

98. Status epilepticus is characterized by:
    A) generalized seizures that last less than 5 minutes.
    B) an absence seizure that is not preceded by an aura.
    C) profound tachycardia and total muscle flaccidity.
    D) prolonged seizures without a return of consciousness.

99. Facial injuries should be identified and treated as soon as possible because:
    A) of the risk for airway problems.
    B) bleeding must be controlled early.
    C) the spine may be injured as well.
    D) swelling may mask hidden injuries.

100. Asthma is caused by a response of the:
    A) immune system.
    B) endocrine system.
    C) respiratory system.
    D) cardiovascular system.

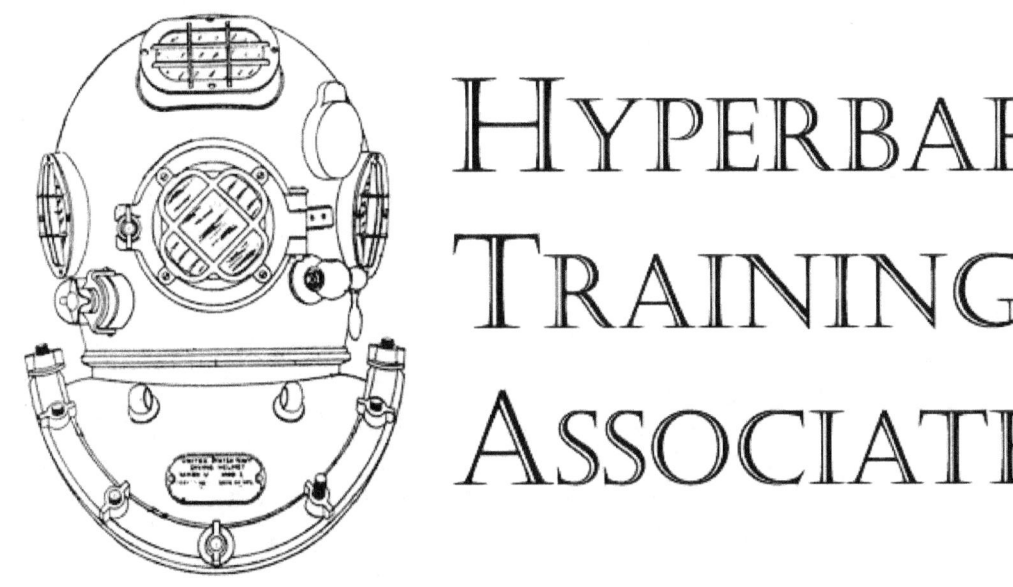

Hyperbaric Training Associates

Diver Medic

Oxygen Treatment Table

Tender Bailouts

www.divermedicaltechnician.com

Tender/Medic Oxygen Bailout USN Table 5			
Depth	Time	Deco Stops (min)	
(fsw)	(hr:min)	20 fsw	10 fsw
60	0:50		No-Deco
55	0:55		1
50	1:00		4
45	1:05		5
40	1:10		6
35	1:15		7
30	1:20		7
30	1:25		7
30	1:30		6
30	1:35		6
30	1:40		6
30	1:45		6
30	1:50		6
25	1:55		5
20	2:00		5
15*	2:05		5
10	2:10	Do Not Bailout Finish Run with Tender On O2	
* Tender/Medic Goes on Oxygen			

Tender/Medic Oxygen Bailout USN Table 6			
Depth	Time	Deco Stops (min)	
(fsw)	(hr:min)	20 fsw	10 fsw
60	0:50		No-Deco
60	0:55		2
60	1:00		5
60	1:05		7
60	1:10		10
60	1:15		12
60	1:20		14
55	1:25		16
50	1:30		17
45	1:35		17
40	1:40		18
35	1:45		17
30	1:50		17
30	1:55		16
30	2:00		16
30	2:05		16
30	2:10		16
30	2:15		16
30	2:20		16
30	2:25		16
30	2:30		16
30	2:35		16
30	2:40		16
30	2:45		16
30	2:50		16
30	2:55		16
30	3:00		16
30	3:05		16
30	3:10		16
30	3:15		16
30	3:20		16
30	3:25		16
30	3:30		16
30	3:35		16
30	3:40		16
30	3:45		16
30	3:50		16
30	3:55		16
30	4:00		16
30	4:05		16

Depth	Time	Deco Stops (min)	
(fsw)	(hr:min)	20 fsw	10 fsw
30	4:10		16
30	4:15		16
30*	4:20		16
30	3:00		16
30	3:05		16
30	3:10		16
30	3:15		16
30	3:20		16
30	3:25		16
30	3:30		16
30	3:35		16
30	3:40		16
30	3:45		16
30	3:50		16
30	3:55		16
30	4:00		16
30	4:05		16
30	4:10		16
30	4:15		16
30*	4:20		16
25	4:25		16
20	4:30		16
15	4:35		15
10	4:40		
		Do Not Bailout	
* Tender/Medic Goes on Oxygen			

Tender/Medic Oxygen Bailout			
USN Table 6 with 1 Extension @ 60fsw			
Depth (fsw)	Time (hr:min)	Deco Stops (min) 20 fsw	10 fsw
60	0:50		No-Deco
60	0:55		2
60	1:00		5
60	1:05		7
60	1:10		10
60	1:15		12
60	1:20		14
60	1:25		16
60	1:30		18
60	1:35	1	18
60	1:40	2	19
60	1:45	3	19
55	1:50	4	19
50	1:55	5	20
45	2:00	5	22
40	2:05	5	22
35	2:10	5	23
30	2:15	4	23
30	2:20	3	24
30	2:25	2	25
30	2:30	1	25
30	2:35		26
30	2:40		26
30	2:45		25
30	2:50		25
30	2:55		25
30	3:00		24
30	3:05		24
30	3:10		24
30	3:15		24
30	3:20		23
30	3:25		23
30	3:30		23
30	3:35		23
30	3:40		22
30	3:45		22
30	3:50		22
30	3:55		22
30	4:00		22
30	4:05		22
30	4:10		21
30	4:15		21
30	4:20		21

Depth (fsw)	Time (hr:min)	Deco Stops (min) 20 fsw	10 fsw
30	4:20		21
30	4:25		21
30*	4:30		21
30	4:35		16
30	4:40		12
30	4:45		7
25	4:50	Do Not Bailout Finish Run With Tender on Oxygen	
20	4:55		
15	5:00		
10	5:05		
5	5:10		
0	5:15		
* Tender/Medic Goes on Oxygen			

Tender/Medic Oxygen Bailout			
USN Table 6 with 1 Extension @30fsw			
Depth	Time	Deco Stops (min)	
(fsw)	(hr:min)	20 fsw	10 fsw
60	0:50		No-Deco
60	0:55		2
60	1:00		5
60	1:05		7
60	1:10		10
60	1:15		12
60	1:20		14
55	1:25		16
50	1:30		17
45	1:35		17
40	1:40		18
35	1:45		17
30	1:50		17
30	1:55		16
30	2:00		16
30	2:05		16
30	2:10		16
30	2:15		16
30	2:20		16
30	2:25		16
30	2:30		16
30	2:35		16
30	2:40		16
30	2:45		16
30	2:50		16
30	2:55		16
30	3:00		16
30	3:05		16
30	3:10		16
30	3:15		16
30	3:20		16
30	3:25		16
30	3:30		16
30	3:35		16
30	3:40		16
30	3:45		16
30	3:50		16
30	3:55		16
30	4:00		16
30	4:05		16
30	4:10		16
30	4:15		16
30	4:20		16

Depth	Time	Deco Stops (min)	
(fsw)	(hr:min)	20 fsw	10 fsw
30	4:25		16
30	4:30		16
30	4:35		16
30	4:40		16
30	4:45		16
30	4:50		16
30	4:55		16
30	5:00		16
30	5:05		16
30	5:10		16
30	5:15		17
30*	5:20		17
30	5:25		12
30	5:30		8
30	5:35		3
25	5:40	Do Not Bailout	
20	5:45	Finish Run With	
15	5:50	Tender on Oxygen	
10	5:55		
5	6:00		
0	6:05		
* Tender/Medic Goes on Oxygen			

Tender/Medic Oxygen Bailout			
USN Table 6 with 2 Extensions @30fsw			
Depth	Time	Deco Stops (min)	
(fsw)	(hr:min)	20 fsw	10 fsw
60	0:50		No-Deco
60	0:55		2
60	1:00		5
60	1:05		7
60	1:10		10
60	1:15		12
60	1:20		14
55	1:25		16
50	1:30		17
45	1:35		17
40	1:40		18
35	1:45		17
30	1:50		17
30	1:55		16
30	2:00		16
30	2:05		16
30	2:10		16
30	2:15		16
30	2:20		16
30	2:25		16
30	2:30		16
30	2:35		16
30	2:40		16
30	2:45		16
30	2:50		16
30	2:55		16
30	3:00		16
30	3:05		16
30	3:10		16
30	3:15		16
30	3:20		16
30	3:25		16
30	3:30		16
30	3:35		16
30	3:40		16
30	3:45		16
30	3:50		16
30	3:55		16
30	4:00		16
30	4:05		16
30	4:10		16
30	4:15		16
30	4:20		16

Depth	Time	Deco Stops (min)	
(fsw)	(hr:min)	20 fsw	10 fsw
30	4:25		16
30	4:30		16
30	4:35		16
30	4:40		16
30	4:45		16
30	4:50		16
30	4:55		16
30	5:00		16
30	5:05		16
30	5:10		16
30	5:15		17
30	5:20		17
30	5:25		17
30	5:30		17
30	5:35		18
30	5:40		18
30	5:45		18
30	5:50		18
30	5:55		19
30	6:00		19
30	6:05		19
30	6:10		19
30	6:15		20
30	6:20		20
30	6:25		20
30	6:30		20
30*	6:35		21
30	6:40		16
30	6:45		12
30	6:50		7
25	6:55	Do Not Bailout Finish Run With Tender on Oxygen	
20	7:00		
15	7:05		
10	7:10		
5	7:15		
0	7:20		
* Tender/Medic Goes on Oxygen			

Tender/Medic Oxygen Bailout
USN Table 6 with
1 Extension @ 60fsw 2 Extensions @ 30fsw

Depth (fsw)	Time (hr:min)	Deco Stops (min) 20 fsw	Deco Stops (min) 10 fsw
60	0:50		No-Deco
60	0:55		2
60	1:00		5
60	1:05		7
60	1:10		10
60	1:15		12
60	1:20		14
60	1:25		16
60	1:30		18
60	1:35	1	18
60	1:40	2	19
60	1:45	3	19
55	1:50	4	19
50	1:55	5	20
45	2:00	5	22
40	2:05	5	22
35	2:10	5	23
30	2:15	4	23
30	2:20	3	24
30	2:25	2	25
30	2:30	1	25
30	2:35		26
30	2:40		26
30	2:45		25
30	2:50		25
30	2:55		25
30	3:00		24
30	3:05		24
30	3:10		24
30	3:15		24
30	3:20		23
30	3:25		23
30	3:30		23
30	3:35		23
30	3:40		22
30	3:45		22
30	3:50		22
30	3:55		22
30	4:00		22
30	4:05		22
30	4:10		21
30	4:15		21
30	4:20		21
30	4:25		21
30	4:30		21
30	4:35		21
30	4:40		21
30	4:45		21
30	4:50		21
30	4:55		22
30	5:00		22
30	5:05		22
30	5:10		22
30	5:15		22
30	5:20		22
30	5:25		23
30	5:30		23
30	5:35		23
30	5:40		23
30	5:45		23
30	5:50		23
30	5:55		23
30	6:00		24
30	6:05		24
30	6:10		24
30	6:15		24
30	6:20		24
30	6:25		24
30	6:30		24
30	6:35		24
30	6:40		25
30	6:45		25
30	6:50		25
30*	6:55		25
30	7:00		20
30	7:05		16
30	7:10		11
30	7:15		7
25	7:20	Do Not Bailout Finish Run With Tender on Oxygen	
20	7:25		
15	7:30		
10	7:35		
5	7:40		
0	7:45		

* Tender/Medic Goes on Oxygen

150

Tender/Medic Oxygen Bailout USN Table 6 with 2 Extensions @ 60fsw			
Depth (fsw)	Time (hr:min)	Deco Stops (min)	
		20 fsw	10 fsw
60	0:50		No-Deco
60	0:55		2
60	1:00		5
60	1:05		7
60	1:10		10
60	1:15		12
60	1:20		14
60	1:25		16
60	1:30		18
60	1:35	1	18
60	1:40	2	19
60	1:45	3	19
60	1:50	5	19
60	1:55	6	20
60	2:00	7	22
60	2:05	8	23
60	2:10	9	24
55	2:15	10	25
50	2:20	10	26
45	2:25	10	27
40	2:30	9	28
35	2:35	9	28
30	2:40	7	30
30	2:45	6	30
30	2:50	5	30
30	2:55	4	31
30	3:00	3	31
30	3:05	2	31
30	3:10	1	32
30	3:15		32
30	3:20		32
30	3:25		31
30	3:30		31
30	3:35		30
30	3:40		30
30	3:45		29
30	3:50		29
30	3:55		28
30	4:00		28
30	4:05		28
30	4:10		28
30	4:15		28

Depth (fsw)	Time (hr:min)	Deco Stops (min)	
		20 fsw	10 fsw
30	4:20		28
30	4:25		28
30	4:30		28
30	4:35		28
30	4:40		28
30	4:45		28
30*	4:50		28
30	4:55		24
30	5:00		19
30	5:05		15
30	5:10		11
25	5:15	Do Not Bailout Finish Run With Tender on Oxygen	
20	5:20		
15	5:25		
10	5:30		
5	5:35		
0	5:40		
* Tender/Medic Goes on Oxygen			

151

Tender/Medic Oxygen Bailout USN Table 6 with 1 Extension @ 60fsw 1 Extension @ 30fsw			
Depth (fsw)	Time (hr:min)	Deco Stops (min) 20 fsw	10 fsw
60	0:50		No-Deco
60	0:55		2
60	1:00		5
60	1:05		7
60	1:10		10
60	1:15		12
60	1:20		14
60	1:25		16
60	1:30		18
60	1:35	1	18
60	1:40	2	19
60	1:45	3	19
55	1:50	4	19
50	1:55	5	20
45	2:00	5	22
40	2:05	5	22
35	2:10	5	23
30	2:15	4	23
30	2:20	3	24
30	2:25	2	25
30	2:30	1	25
30	2:35		26
30	2:40		26
30	2:45		25
30	2:50		25
30	2:55		25
30	3:00		24
30	3:05		24
30	3:10		24
30	3:15		24
30	3:20		23
30	3:25		23
30	3:30		23
30	3:35		23
30	3:40		22
30	3:45		22
30	3:50		22
30	3:55		22
30	4:00		22
30	4:05		22
30	4:10		21
30	4:15		21
30	4:20		21
30	4:25		21
30	4:30		21
30	4:35		21
30	4:40		21
30	4:45		21
30	4:50		21
30	4:55		22
30	5:00		22
30	5:05		22
30	5:10		22
30	5:15		22
30	5:20		22
30	5:25		23
30	5:30		23
30	5:35		23
30	5:40		23
30*	5:45		23
30	5:50		19
30	5:55		14
30	6:00		10
25	6:05	Do Not Bailout Finish Run With Tender on Oxygen	
20	6:10		
15	6:15		
10	6:20		
5	6:25		
0	6:30		
* Tender/Medic Goes on Oxygen			

Tender/Medic Oxygen Bailout
USN Table 6 with
2 Extensions @ 60fsw 1 Extension @ 30fsw

Depth (fsw)	Time (hr:min)	Deco Stops (min) 20 fsw	Deco Stops (min) 10 fsw
60	0:50		No-Deco
60	0:55		2
60	1:00		5
60	1:05		7
60	1:10		10
60	1:15		12
60	1:20		14
60	1:25		16
60	1:30		18
60	1:35	1	18
60	1:40	2	19
60	1:45	3	19
60	1:50	5	19
60	1:55	6	20
60	2:00	7	22
60	2:05	8	23
60	2:10	9	24
55	2:15	10	25
50	2:20	10	26
45	2:25	10	27
40	2:30	9	28
35	2:35	9	28
30	2:40	7	30
30	2:45	6	30
30	2:50	5	30
30	2:55	4	31
30	3:00	3	31
30	3:05	2	31
30	3:10	1	32
30	3:15		32
30	3:20		32
30	3:25		31
30	3:30		31
30	3:35		30
30	3:40		30
30	3:45		29
30	3:50		29
30	3:55		28
30	4:00		28
30	4:05		28
30	4:10		28
30	4:15		28
30	4:20		28
30	4:25		28
30	4:30		28
30	4:35		28
30	4:40		28
30	4:45		28
30	4:50		28
30	4:55		28
30	5:00		28
30	5:05		28
30	5:10		28
30	5:15		29
30	5:20		29
30	5:25		29
30	5:30		29
30	5:35		29
30	5:40		29
30	5:45		29
30	5:50		29
30	5:55		29
30	6:00		29
30*	6:05		29
30	6:10		24
30	6:15		20
30	6:20		15
30	6:25		11
25	6:30	Do Not Bailout Finish Run With Tender on Oxygen	
20	6:35		
15	6:40		
10	6:45		
5	6:50		
0	6:55		

* Tender/Medic Goes on Oxygen

153

Tender/Medic Oxygen Bailout							
USN Table 6 with							
2 Extensions @ 60fsw 2 Extension @ 30fsw							
Depth	Time	Deco Stops (min)		Depth	Time	Deco Stops (min)	
(fsw)	(hr:min)	20 fsw	10 fsw	(fsw)	(hr:min)	20 fsw	10 fsw
60	0:50		No-Deco	30	4:35		28
60	0:55		2	30	4:40		28
60	1:00		5	30	4:45		28
60	1:05		7	30	4:50		28
60	1:10		10	30	4:55		28
60	1:15		12	30	5:00		28
60	1:20		14	30	5:05		28
60	1:25		16	30	5:10		28
60	1:30		18	30	5:15		29
60	1:35	1	18	30	5:20		29
60	1:40	2	19	30	5:25		29
60	1:45	3	19	30	5:30		29
60	1:50	5	19	30	5:35		29
60	1:55	6	20	30	5:40		29
60	2:00	7	22	30	5:45		29
60	2:05	8	23	30	5:50		29
60	2:10	9	24	30	5:55		29
55	2:15	10	25	30	6:00		29
50	2:20	10	26	30	6:05		29
45	2:25	10	27	30	6:10		29
40	2:30	9	28	30	6:15		29
35	2:35	9	28	30	6:20		29
30	2:40	7	30	30	6:25		29
30	2:45	6	30	30	6:30		29
30	2:50	5	30	30	6:35		29
30	2:55	4	31	30	6:40		29
30	3:00	3	31	30	6:45		29
30	3:05	2	31	30	6:50		29
30	3:10	1	32	30	6:55		30
30	3:15		32	30	7:00		30
30	3:20		32	30	7:05		30
30	3:25		31	30*	7:10		31
30	3:30		31	30	7:15		26
30	3:35		30	30	7:20		24
30	3:40		30	30	7:25		17
30	3:45		29	30	7:30		12
30	3:50		29	30	7:35		8
30	3:55		28	30	7:40		4
30	4:00		28	25	7:45	Do Not Bailout	
30	4:05		28	20	7:50	Finish Run With	
30	4:10		28	15	7:55	Tender on Oxygen	
30	4:15		28	10	8:00		
30	4:20		28	5	8:05		
30	4:25		28	0	8:10		
30	4:30		28	* Tender/Medic Goes on Oxygen			

Tender/Medic Oxygen Bailout

Comex 30							Comex 30						
Time		Depth	Deco Stops (min)				Time		Depth	Deco Stops (min)			
(hr:min)	(hr:min)	(fsw)	40 fsw	30 fsw	20 fsw	10 fsw	(hr:min)	(hr:min)	(fsw)	40 fsw	30 fsw	20 fsw	10 fsw
0:00	0:07	0-100	No Deco				4:22	4:27	40		7	43	67
0:07	0:17	100	No Deco				4:27	4:32	40		6	44	67
0:17	0:22	100				2	4:32	4:37	40		6	43	69
0:22	0:27	100			1	4	4:37	4:42	40		5	44	69
0:27	0:32	100			2	10	4:42	4:47	40		4	45	69
0:32	0:37	100			5	13	4:47	4:52	40		4	44	70
0:37	0:42	100			7	17	4:52			No Bailout - Finish Table			
0:42	0:47	100		1	9	18							
0:47	0:52	100-97		3	11	18							
0:52	0:57	97-93		4	13	19							
0:57	1:02	93-90		4	16	22							
1:02	1:07	90-87		5	18	23							
1:07	1:12	87-83		5	19	26							
1:12	1:17	83-80		7	19	28							
1:17	1:22	80		9	19	29							
1:22	1:27	80		10	19	31							
1:27	1:32	80		11	19	33							
1:32	1:37	80		12	20	34							
1:37	1:42	80		13	22	34							
1:42	1:47	80	1	17	19	34							
1:47	1:52	80-77	2	17	20	36							
1:52	1:57	77-73	2	17	22	37							
1:57	2:02	73-70	3	17	23	38							
2:02	2:07	70-67	3	17	24	40							
2:07	2:12	67-63	3	17	25	41							
2:12	2:17	63-60	3	17	26	42							
2:17	2:22	60	2	17	27	43							
2:22	2:27	60	2	17	28	44							
2:27	2:32	60	1	14	32	45							
2:32	2:37	60	1	13	33	47							
2:37	2:42	60	1	13	34	47							
2:42	2:47	60	1	13	34	49							
2:47	2:52	60		14	35	51							
2:52	2:57	60		15	35	52							
2:57	3:02	60		15	35	55							
3:02	3:07	60		16	34	57							
3:07	3:12	60		16	35	58							
3:12	3:17	60		16	36	59							
3:17	3:22	60-57		16	36	60							
3:22	3:27	57-53		16	37	60							
3:27	3:32	53-50		16	38	61							
3:32	3:37	50-47		16	38	62							
3:37	3:42	47-43		15	39	62							
3:42	3:47	43-40		14	40	63							
3:47	3:52	40		13	40	64							
3:52	3:57	40		12	41	64							
3:57	4:02	40		11	41	65							
4:02	4:07	40		10	42	65							
4:07	4:12	40		10	41	66							
4:12	4:17	40		9	42	66							
4:17	4:22	40		8	43	66							

155

Tender/Medic Oxygen Bailout					
Comex 30 with Prior Start of USN 6					
Time		Depth	Deco Stops (min)		
(hr:min)	(hr:min)	(fsw)	40 fsw	30 fsw	20 fsw	10 fsw
0:00	0:50	(USN 6 @60fsw)				
0:50	0:55	60-100				12
0:55	1:00	100			2	16
1:00	1:05	100			5	19
1:05	1:10	100			10	18
1:10	1:15	100		1	13	19
1:15	1:20	100		3	15	21
1:20	1:25	100		4	17	24
1:25	1:30	100		5	20	26
1:30	1:35	100	1	11	15	29
1:35	1:40	100-97	2	12	16	31
1:40	1:45	97-93	2	14	16	33
1:45	1:50	93-90	2	16	16	34
1:50	1:55	90-87	3	17	17	34
1:55	2:00	87-83	4	17	19	34
2:00	2:05	83-80	4	17	21	36
2:05	2:10	80	5	17	22	38
2:10	2:15	80	6	17	23	39
2:15	2:20	80	6	17	25	41
2:20	2:25	80	7	17	26	42
2:25	2:30	80	8	17	27	43
2:30	2:35	80	8	17	29	44
2:35	2:40	80-77	8	19	28	46
2:40	2:45	77-73	9	19	28	48
2:45	2:50	73-70	9	20	28	50
2:50	2:55	70-67	8	21	29	52
2:55	3:00	67-63	8	22	28	54
3:00	3:05	63-60	7	23	29	55
3:05	3:10	60	7	23	29	57
3:10	3:15	60	6	24	29	59
3:15	3:20	60	6	24	30	60
3:20	3:25	60	5	25	31	60

Time (hr:min)	(hr:min)	Depth (fsw)	Deco Stops (min)			
			40 fsw	30 fsw	20 fsw	10 fsw
3:25	3:30	60	5	25	32	61
3:30	3:35	60	4	26	33	62
3:35	3:40	60	4	27	33	63
3:40	3:45	60	3	28	34	63
3:45	3:50	60	3	28	34	65
3:50	3:55	60	2	29	35	65
3:55	4:00	60	2	29	36	66
4:00	4:05	60	2	29	37	66
4:05	4:10	60-57	1	23	44	67
4:10	4:15	57-53		24	44	68
4:15	4:20	53-50		23	45	69
4:20	4:25	50-47		23	45	69
4:25	4:30	47-43		22	46	69
4:30	4:35	43-40		21	46	71
4:35	4:40	40		20	47	71
4:40	4:45	40		19	47	72
4:45	4:50	40		17	48	74
4:50	4:55	40		16	48	75
4:55	5:00	40		15	49	76
5:00	5:05	40		14	49	77
5:05	5:10	40		13	50	78
5:10	5:15	40		12	50	79
5:15	To End of Run		Do Not Bailout - Finish Run as Planned			

Tender/Medic Oxygen Bailout								
USN Table 6A								
Depth	Time	Decompression Stops						
(fsw)	(hr:min)	Air		Oxygen				
		70 fsw	60 fsw	50 fsw	40 fsw	30 fsw	20 fsw	10 fsw
165	0:05	No Decompression Required						
165	0:10						2	2
165	0:15				2		2	4
165	0:20			2	2		4	12
165	0:25		2	2	2	2	6	18
165	0:30	2	2	2	2	6	10	18
165-60	0:34		1	2	2	6	10	18
60	0:39				4	5	12	18
60	0:44				2	6	13	19
60	0:49				1	5	15	21
60	0:54					6	15	23
60	0:59					6	16	23
60	1:04					6	16	25
60	1:09					6	16	27
60	1:14					6	16	28
60	1:19					7	15	30
60	1:24					7	16	30
60	1:29					7	16	32
60	1:34					7	16	33
60	1:39					7	16	34
60	1:44					8	16	34
60	1:49					8	17	35
55	1:53					8	18	34
50	1:59					7	20	34
45	2:04					7	20	35
40	2:09					6	20	36
35	2:14					5	26	36
30	2:19					3	22	37
30	2:24					1	22	38
30	2:29						22	39
30	2:34						21	39
30	2:39						20	40

Depth (fsw)	Time (hr:min)	Decompression Stops						
		Air		Oxygen				
		70 fsw	60 fsw	50 fsw	40 fsw	30 fsw	20 fsw	10 fsw
30	2:44						19	40
30	2:49						18	41
30	2:54						17	41
30	2:59						16	42
30	3:04						15	42
30	3:09						14	43
30	3:14						13	43
30	3:19						12	44
30	3:24						12	43
30	3:29						11	44
30	3:34						10	44
30	3:39						9	45
30	3:44						8	46
30	3:49						8	45
30	3:54						7	46
30	3:59						6	47
30	4:04*						6	47
30	4:09						5	48
30	4:14						4	43
30	4:19						4	39
30	4:24							34
30	4:29							30
30	4:34							26
30	4:39							21
30	4:44							17
30	4:49							13
25	4:54							12
20	4:59							12
15	5:04			Do Not Bailout				
10	5:09			Finish Run With				
5	5:14			Tender on Oxygen				
0				* Tender/Medic Goes on Oxygen				

159

APPENDIX 5A
Neurological Examination

5A-1 INTRODUCTION

This appendix provides guidance on evaluating diving accidents prior to treatment. Figure 5A-1a is a guide aimed at non-medical personnel for recording essential details and conducting a neurological examination. Copies of this form should be readily available. While its use is not mandatory, it provides a useful aid for gathering information.

5A-2 INITIAL ASSESSMENT OF DIVING INJURIES

When using the form in Figure 5A-1a, the initial assessment must gather the necessary information for proper evaluation of the accident.

When a diver reports with a medical complaint, a history of the case shall be compiled. This history should include facts ranging from the dive profile to progression of the medical problem. If available, review the diver's Health Record and completed Diving Chart or Diving Log to aid in the examination. A few key questions can help determine a preliminary diagnosis and any immediate treatment needed. If the preliminary diagnosis shows the need for immediate recompression, proceed with recompression. Complete the examination when the patient stabilizes at treatment depth. Typical questions should include the following:

1. What is the problem/symptom? If the only symptom is pain:

    a. Describe the pain:
       - Sharp
       - Dull
       - Throbbing

    b. Is the pain localized, or hard to pinpoint?

2. Has the patient made a dive recently?

3. What was the dive profile?

    a. What was the depth of the dive?

    b. What was the bottom time?

    c. What dive rig was used?

    d. What type of work was performed?

    e. Did anything unusual occur during the dive?

4. How many dives has the patient made in the last 24 hours?

    a. Chart profile(s) of any other dive(s).

5. Were the symptoms first noted before, during, or after the dive? If after the dive, how long after surfacing?

6. If during the dive, did the patient notice the symptom while descending, on the bottom, or during ascent?

7. Has the symptom either increased or decreased in intensity since first noticed?

8. Have any additional symptoms developed since the first one?

9. Has the patient ever had a similar symptom?

10. Has the patient ever suffered from decompression sickness or gas embolism in the past?

    a. Describe this symptom in relation to the prior incident if applicable.

11. Does the patient have any concurrent medical conditions that might explain the symptoms?

To aid in the evaluation, review the diver's Health Record, including a baseline neurological examination, if available, and completed Diving Chart or Diving Log, if they are readily available.

5A-3 NEUROLOGICAL ASSESSMENT

There are various ways to perform a neurological examination. The quickest information pertinent to the diving injury is obtained by directing the initial examination toward the symptomatic areas of the body. These concentrate on the motor, sensory, and coordination functions. If this examination is normal, the most productive information is obtained by performing a complete examination of the following:

1. Mental status
2. Coordination
3. Motor
4. Cranial nerves
5. Sensory
6. Deep tendon reflexes

The following procedures are adequate for preliminary examination. Figure 5A-1a can be used to record the results of the examination.

NEUROLOGICAL EXAMINATION CHECKLIST

(Sheet 1 of 2)

(See text of Appendix 5A for examination procedures and definitions of terms.)

Patient's Name: _____ Date/Time: _____

Describe pain/numbness: _____

_____

HISTORY

Type of dive last performed: _____ Depth: _____ How long: _____

Number of dives in last 24 hours: _____

Was symptom noticed before, during or after the dive? _____

If during, was it while descending, on the bottom or ascending? _____

Has symptom increased or decreased since it was first noticed? _____

Have any other symptoms occurred since the first one was noticed? _____

Describe: _____

Has patient ever had a similar symptom before? _____ When: _____

_____

MENTAL STATUS/STATE OF CONSCIOUSNESS

_____

_____

COORDINATION

Walk: _____

Heel-to Toe: _____

Romberg: _____

Finger-to-Nose: _____

Heel Shin Slide: _____

Rapid Movement: _____

CRANIAL NERVES

Sense of Smell (I): _____

Vision/Visual Fld (II): _____

Eye Movements, Pupils (III, IV, VI): _____

Facial Sensation, Chewing (V): _____

Facial Expression Muscles (VII): _____

Hearing (VIII): _____

Upper Mouth, Throat Sensation (IX): _____

Gag & Voice (X): _____

Shoulder Shrug (XI): _____

Tongue (XII): _____

STRENGTH (Grade 0 to 5)

UPPER BODY

Deltoids   L _____ R _____
Latissimus   L _____ R _____
Biceps   L _____ R _____
Triceps   L _____ R _____
Forearms   L _____ R _____
Hand   L _____ R _____

LOWER BODY

HIPS

Flexion   L _____ R _____
Extension   L _____ R _____
Abduction   L _____ R _____
Adduction   L _____ R _____

KNEES

Flexion   L _____ R _____
Extension   L _____ R _____

ANKLES

Dorsiflexion   L _____ R _____
Plantarflexion L _____ R _____

TOES

L _____ R _____

Figure 5A-1a. Neurological Examination Checklist (sheet 1 of 2).

NEUROLOGICAL EXAMINATION CHECKLIST
(Sheet 2 of 2)

REFLEXES

(Grade: Normal, Hypoactive, Hyperactive, Absent)

Biceps	L _____	R _____
Triceps	L _____	R _____
Knees	L _____	R _____
Ankles	L _____	R _____

Sensory Examination for Skin Sensation
(Use diagram to record location of sensory abnormalities – numbness, tingling, etc.)

LOCATION

Indicate results as follows:

|||| Painful Area

═══ Decreased Sensation

COMMENTS

_____
_____
_____
_____
_____
_____
_____
_____

Examination Performed by: _____

Figure 5A-1b. Neurological Examination Checklist (sheet 2 of 2).

5A-3.1 **Mental Status.** This is best determined when you first see the patient and is characterized by his alertness, orientation, and thought process. Obtain a good history, including the dive profile, present symptoms, and how these symptoms have changed since onset. The patient's response to this questioning and that during the neurological examination will give you a great deal of information about his mental status. It is important to determine if the patient knows the time and place, and can recognize familiar people and understands what is happening. Is the patient's mood appropriate?

Next the examiner may determine if the patient's memory is intact by questioning the patient. The questions asked should be reasonable, and you must know the answer to the questions you ask. Questions such as the following may be helpful:

- What is your commanding officer's name?
- What did you have for lunch?

Finally, if a problem does arise in the mental status evaluation, the examiner may choose to assess the patient's cognitive function more fully. Cognitive function is an intellectual process by which one becomes aware of, perceives, or comprehends ideas and involves all aspects of perception, thinking, reasoning, and remembering. Some suggested methods of assessing this function are:

- The patient should be asked to remember something. An example would be "red ball, green tree, and couch." Inform him that later in the examination you will ask him to repeat this information.
- The patient should be asked to spell a word, such as "world," backwards.
- The patient should be asked to count backwards from 100 by sevens.
- The patient should be asked to recall the information he was asked to remember at the end of the examination.

5A-3.2 **Coordination (Cerebellar/Inner Ear Function).** A good indicator of muscle strength and general coordination is to observe how the patient walks. A normal gait indicates that many muscle groups and general brain functions are normal. More thorough examination involves testing that concentrates on the brain and inner ear. In conducting these tests, both sides of the body shall be tested and the results shall be compared. These tests include:

1. **Heel-to-Toe Test.** The tandem walk is the standard "drunk driver" test. While looking straight ahead, the patient must walk a straight line, placing the heel of one foot directly in front of the toes of the opposite foot. Signs to look for and consider deficits include:

    a. Does the patient limp?

    b. Does the patient stagger or fall to one side?

2. **Romberg Test.** With eyes closed, the patient stands with feet together and arms extended to the front, palms up. Note whether the patient can maintain his balance or if he immediately falls to one side. Some examiners recommend giving the patient a small shove from either side with the fingertips.

3. **Finger-to-Nose Test.** The patient stands with eyes closed and head back, arms extended to the side. Bending the arm at the elbow, the patient touches his nose with an extended forefinger, alternating arms. An extension of this test is to have the patient, with eyes open, alternately touch his nose with his fingertip and then touch the fingertip of the examiner. The examiner will change the position of his fingertip each time the patient touches his nose. In this version, speed is not important, but accuracy is.

4. **Heel-Shin Slide Test.** While standing, the patient touches the heel of one foot to the knee of the opposite leg, foot pointing forward. While maintaining this contact, he runs his heel down the shin to the ankle. Each leg should be tested.

5. **Rapid Alternating Movement Test.** The patient slaps one hand on the palm of the other, alternating palm up and then palm down. Any exercise requiring rapidly changing movement, however, will suffice. Again, both sides should be tested.

5A-3.3 **Cranial Nerves.** The cranial nerves are the 12 pairs of nerves emerging from the cranial cavity through various openings in the skull. Beginning with the most anterior (front) on the brain stem, they are appointed Roman numerals. An isolated cranial nerve lesion is an unusual finding in decompression sickness or gas embolism, but deficits occasionally occur and you should test for abnormalities. The cranial nerves must be quickly assessed as follows:

I. **Olfactory.** The olfactory nerve, which provides our sense of smell, is usually not tested.

II. **Optic.** The optic nerve is for vision. It functions in the recognition of light and shade and in the perception of objects. This test should be completed one eye at a time to determine whether the patient can read. Ask the patient if he has any blurring of vision, loss of vision, spots in the visual field, or peripheral vision loss (tunnel vision). More detailed testing can be done by standing in front of the patient and asking him to cover one eye and look straight at you. In a plane midway between yourself and the patient, slowly bring your fingertip in turn from above, below, to the right, and to the left of the direction of gaze until the patient can see it. Compare this with the earliest that you can see it with the equivalent eye. If a deficit is present, roughly map out the positions of the blind spots by passing the finger tip across the visual field.

III. **Oculomotor, (IV.) Trochlear, (VI.) Abducens.** These three nerves control eye movements. All three nerves can be tested by having the patient's eyes follow the examiner's finger in all four directions (quadrants) and then in towards the tip of the nose (giving a "crossed-eyed" look). The oculomotor nerve can be further tested by shining a light into one eye at a time. In a normal response, the pupils of both eyes will constrict.

V. Trigeminal. The Trigeminal Nerve governs sensation of the forehead and face and the clenching of the jaw. It also supplies the muscle of the ear (tensor tympani) necessary for normal hearing. Sensation is tested by lightly stroking the forehead, face, and jaw on each side with a finger or wisp of cotton wool.

VII. Facial. The Facial Nerve controls the face muscles. It stimulates the scalp, forehead, eyelids, muscles of facial expression, cheeks, and jaw. It is tested by having the patient smile, show his teeth, whistle, wrinkle his forehead, and close his eyes tightly. The two sides should perform symmetrically. Symmetry of the nasolabial folds (lines from nose to outside corners of the mouth) should be observed.

VIII. Acoustic. The Acoustic Nerve controls hearing and balance. Test this nerve by whispering to the patient, rubbing your fingers together next to the patient's ears, or putting a tuning fork near the patient's ears. Compare this against the other ear.

IX. Glossopharyngeal. The Glossopharyngeal Nerves transmit sensation from the upper mouth and throat area. It supplies the sensory component of the gag reflex and constriction of the pharyngeal wall when saying "aah." Test this nerve by touching the back of the patient's throat with a tongue depressor. This should cause a gagging response. This nerve is normally not tested.

X. Vagus. The Vagus Nerve has many functions, including control of the roof of the mouth and vocal cords. The examiner can test this nerve by having the patient say "aah" while watching for the palate to rise. Note the tone of the voice; hoarseness may also indicate vagus nerve involvement.

XI. Spinal Accessory. The Spinal Accessory Nerve controls the turning of the head from side to side and shoulder shrug against resistance. Test this nerve by having the patient turn his head from side to side. Resistance is provided by placing one hand against the side of the patient's head. The examiner should note that an injury to the nerve on one side will cause an inability to turn the head to the opposite side or weakness/absence of the shoulder shrug on the affected side.

XII. Hypoglossal. The Hypoglossal Nerve governs the muscle activity of the tongue. An injury to one of the hypoglossal nerves causes the tongue to twist to that side when stuck out of the mouth.

5A-3.4 **Motor.** A diver with decompression sickness may experience disturbances in the muscle system. The range of symptoms can be from a mild twitching of a muscle to weakness and paralysis. No matter how slight the abnormality, symptoms involving the motor system shall be treated.

5A-3.4.1 **Extremity Strength.** It is common for a diver with decompression illness to experience muscle weakness. Extremity strength testing is divided into two parts: upper body and lower body. All muscle groups should be tested and compared with the corresponding group on the other side, as well as with the examiner. Table 5A-1 describes the extremity strength tests in more detail. Muscle strength is graded (0-5) as follows:

- **(0) Paralysis.** No motion possible.
- **(1) Profound Weakness.** Flicker or trace of muscle contraction.
- **(2) Severe Weakness.** Able to contract muscle but cannot move joint against gravity.
- **(3) Moderate Weakness.** Able to overcome the force of gravity but not the resistance of the examiner.
- **(4) Mild Weakness.** Able to resist slight force of examiner.
- **(5) Normal.** Equal strength bilaterally (both sides) and able to resist examiner.

5A-3.4.1.1 *Upper Extremities.* These muscles are tested with resistance provided by the examiner. The patient should overcome force applied by the examiner that is tailored to the patient's strength. Table 5A-1 describes the extremity strength tests. The six muscle groups tested in the upper extremity are:

1. Deltoids.
2. Latissimus.
3. Biceps.
4. Triceps.
5. Forearm muscles.
6. Hand muscles.

5A-3.4.1.2 *Lower Extremities.* The lower extremity strength is assessed by watching the patient walk on his heels for a short distance and then on his toes. The patient should then walk while squatting ("duck walk"). These tests adequately assess lower extremity strength, as well as balance and coordination. If a more detailed examination of the lower extremity strength is desired, testing should be accomplished at each joint as in the upper arm.

5A-3.4.2 **Muscle Size.** Muscles are visually inspected and felt, while at rest, for size and consistency. Look for symmetry of posture and of muscle contours and outlines. Examine for fine muscle twitching.

5A-3.4.3 **Muscle Tone.** Feel the muscles at rest and the resistance to passive movement. Look and feel for abnormalities in tone such as spasticity, rigidity, or no tone.

5A-3.4.4 **Involuntary Movements.** Inspection may reveal slow, irregular, and jerky movements, rapid contractions, tics, or tremors.

5A-3.5 **Sensory Function.** Common presentations of decompression sickness in a diver that may indicate spinal cord dysfunction are:

Table 5A-1. Extremity Strength Tests.

Test	Procedure
Deltoid Muscles	The patient raises his arm to the side at the shoulder joint. The examiner places a hand on the patient's wrist and exerts a downward force that the patient resists.
Latissimus Group	The patient raises his arm to the side. The examiner places a hand on the underside of the patient's wrist and resists the patient's attempt to lower his arm.
Biceps	The patient bends his arm at the elbow, toward his chest. The examiner then grasps the patient's wrist and exerts a force to straighten the patient's arm.
Triceps	The patient bends his arm at the elbow, toward his chest. The examiner then places his hand on the patient's forearm and the patient tries to straighten his arm.
Forearm Muscles	The patient makes a fist. The examiner grips the patient's fist and resists while the patient tries to bend his wrist upward and downward.
Hand Muscles	• The patient strongly grips the examiner's extended fingers. • The patient extends his hand with the fingers widespread. The examiner grips two of the extended fingers with two of his own fingers and tries to squeeze the patient's two fingers together, noting the patient's strength of resistance.
Lower Extremity Strength	• The patient walks on his heels for a short distance. The patient then turns around and walks back on his toes. • The patient walks while squatting (duck walk). These tests adequately assesses lower extremity strength as well as balance and coordination. If a more detailed examination of lower extremity strength is desired, testing should be accomplished at each joint as in the upper arm.

In the following tests, the patient sits on a solid surface such as a desk, with feet off the floor.

Test	Procedure
Hip Flexion	The examiner places his hand on the patient's thigh to resist as the patient tries to raise his thigh.
Hip Extension	The examiner places his hand on the underside of the patient's thigh to resist as the patient tries to lower his thigh.
Hip Abduction	The patients sits as above, with knees together. The examiner places a hand on the outside of each of the patient's knees to provide resistance. The patient tries to open his knees.
Hip Adduction	The patient sits as above, with knees apart. The examiner places a hand on the inside of each of the patient's knees to provide resistance. The patient tries to bring his knees together.
Knee Extension	The examiner places a hand on the patient's shin to resist as the patient tries to straighten his leg.
Knee Flexion	The examiner places a hand on the back of the patient's lower leg to resist as the patient tries to pull his lower leg to the rear by flexing his knee.
Ankle Dorsiflexion (ability to flex the foot toward the rear)	The examiner places a hand on top of the patient's foot to resist as the patient tries to raise his foot by flexing it at the ankle.
Ankle Plantarflexion (ability to flex the foot downward)	The examiner places a hand on the bottom of the patient's foot to resist as the patient tries to lower his foot by flexing it at the ankle.
Toes	• The patient stands on tiptoes for 15 seconds • The patient flexes his toes with resistance provided by the examiner.

- Pain
- Numbness
- Tingling ("pins-and-needles" feeling; also called paresthesia)

5A-3.5.1 **Sensory Examination.** An examination of the patient's sensory faculties should be performed. Figures 5A-2a and 5A-2b show the dermatomal (sensory) areas of skin sensations that correlate with each spinal cord segment. Note that the dermatomal areas of the trunk run in a circular pattern around the trunk. The dermatomal areas in the arms and legs run in a more lengthwise pattern. In a complete examination, each spinal segment should be checked for loss of sensation.

5A-3.5.2 **Sensations.** Sensations easily recognized by most normal people are sharp/dull discrimination (to perceive as separate) and light touch. It is possible to test pressure, temperature, and vibration in special cases. The likelihood of DCS affecting only one sense, however, is very small.

5A-3.5.3 **Instruments.** An ideal instrument for testing changes in sensation is a sharp object, such as the Wartenberg pinwheel or a common safety pin. Either of these objects must applied at intervals. Avoid scratching or penetrating the skin. It is not the intent of this test to cause pain.

5A-3.5.4 **Testing the Trunk.** Move the pinwheel or other sharp object from the top of the shoulder slowly down the front of the torso to the groin area. Another method is to run it down the rear of the torso to just below the buttocks. The patient should be asked if he feels a sharp point and if he felt it all the time. Test each dermatome by going down the trunk on each side of the body. Test the neck area in similar fashion.

5A-3.5.5 **Testing Limbs.** In testing the limbs, a circular pattern of testing is best. Test each limb in at least three locations, and note any difference in sensation on each side of the body. On the arms, circle the arm at the deltoid, just below the elbow, and at the wrist. In testing the legs, circle the upper thigh, just below the knee, and the ankle.

5A-3.5.6 **Testing the Hands.** The hand is tested by running the sharp object across the back and palm of the hand and then across the fingertips.

5A-3.5.7 **Marking Abnormalities.** If an area of abnormality is found, mark the area as a reference point in assessment. Some examiners use a marking pen to trace the area of decreased or increased sensation on the patient's body. During treatment, these areas are rechecked to determine whether the area is improving. An example of improvement is an area of numbness getting smaller.

5A-3.6 **Deep Tendon Reflexes.** The purpose of the deep tendon reflexes is to determine if the patient's response is normal, nonexistent, hypoactive (deficient), or hyperactive (excessive). The patient's response should be compared to responses the examiner has observed before. Notation should be made of whether the responses are equal bilaterally (both sides) and if the upper and lower reflexes are similar. If any difference in the reflexes is noticed, the patient should be asked if there is a prior

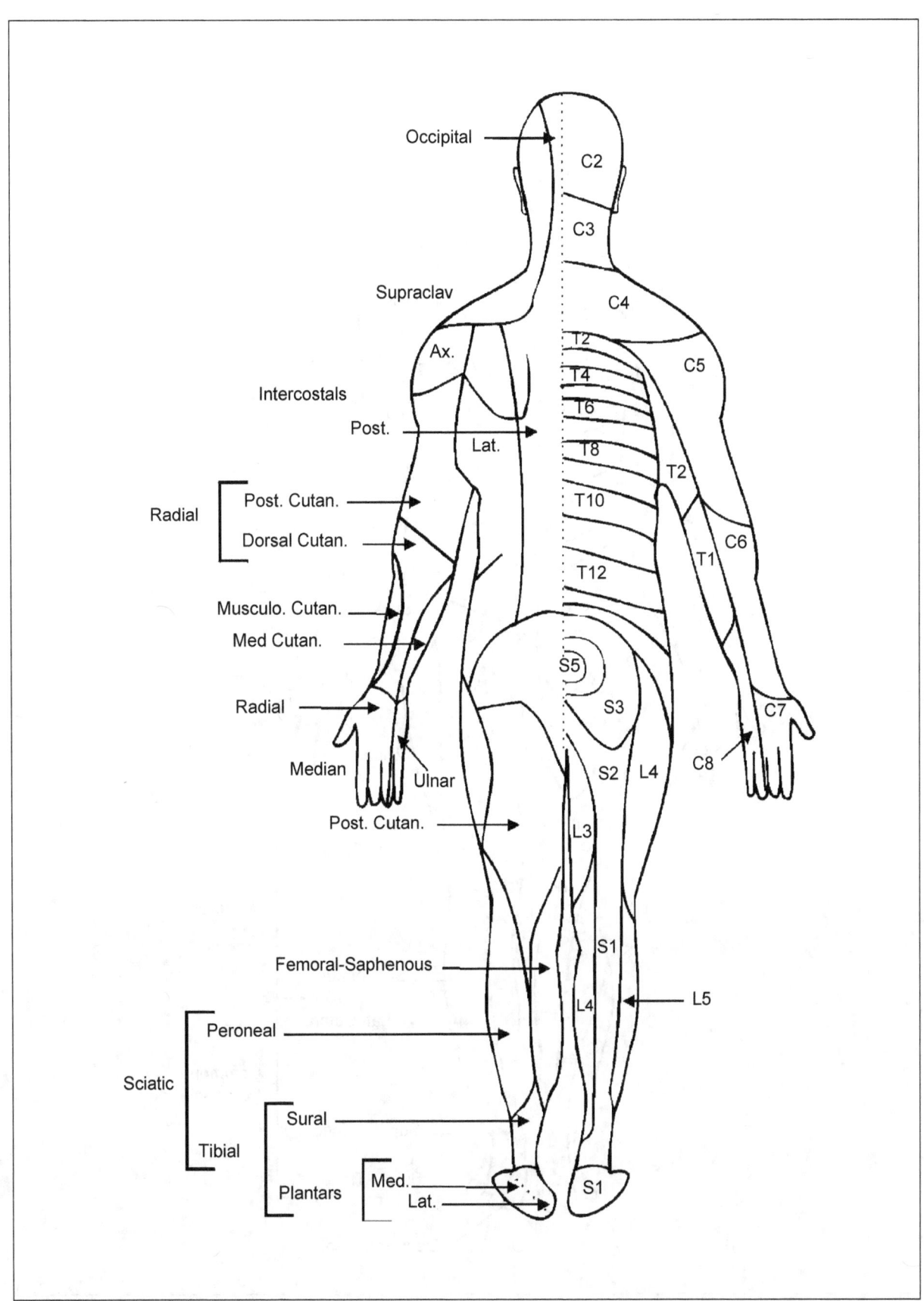

Figure 5A-2a. Dermatomal Areas Correlated to Spinal Cord Segment (sheet 1 of 2).

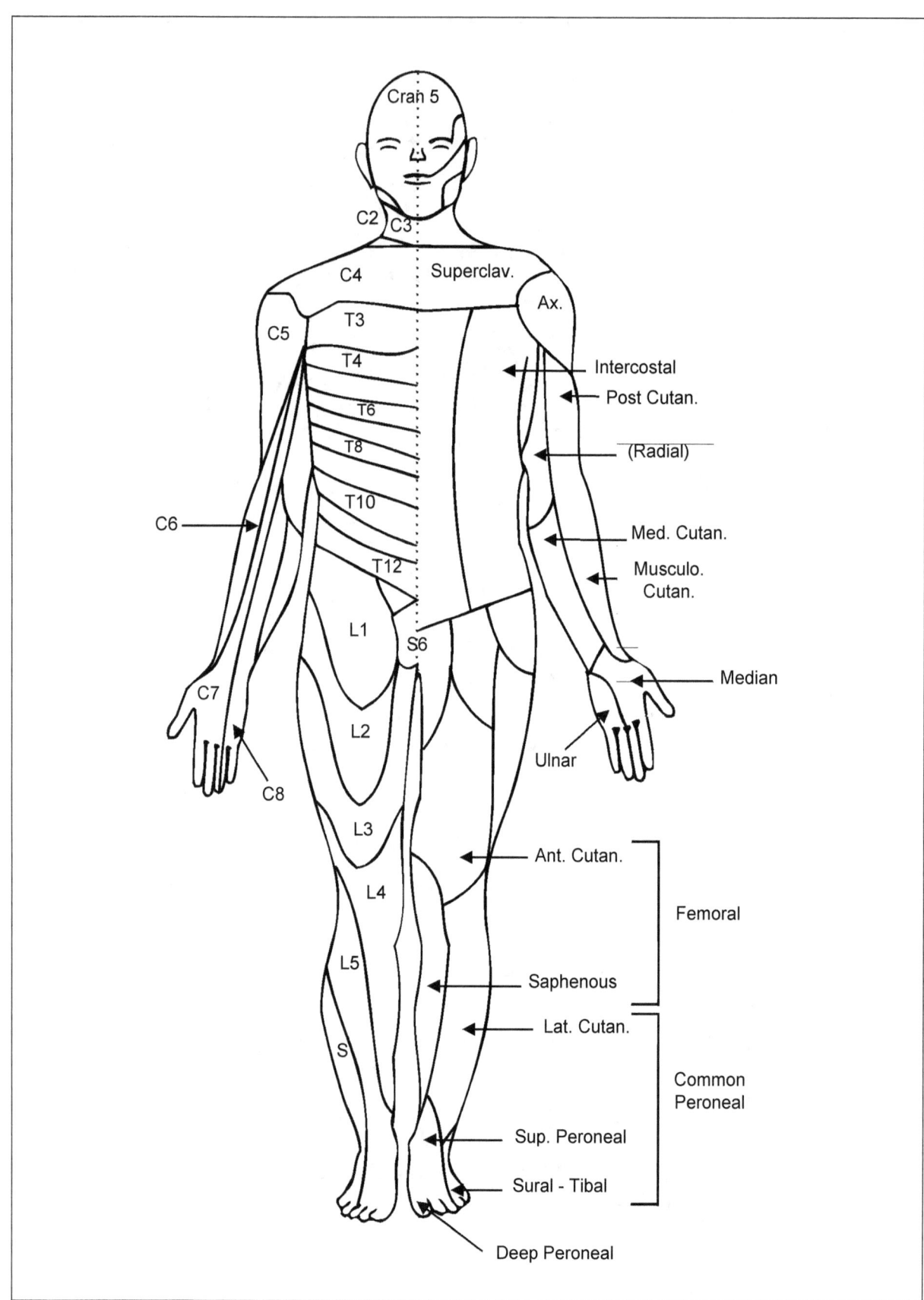

Figure 5A-2b. Dermatomal Areas Correlated to Spinal Cord Segment (sheet 2 of 2).

medical condition or injury that would cause the difference. Isolated differences should not be treated, because it is extremely difficult to get symmetrical responses bilaterally. To get the best response, strike each tendon with an equal, light force, and with sharp, quick taps. Usually, if a deep tendon reflex is abnormal due to decompression sickness, there will be other abnormal signs present. Test the biceps, triceps, knee, and ankle reflexes by striking the tendon as described in Table 5A-2.

Table 5A-2. Reflexes.

Test	Procedure
Biceps	The examiner holds the patient's elbow with the patient's hand resting on the examiner's forearm. The patient's elbow should be slightly bent and his arm relaxed. The examiner places his thumb on the patient's biceps tendon, located in the bend of the patient's elbow. The examiner taps his thumb with the percussion hammer, feeling for the patient's muscle to contract.
Triceps	The examiner supports the patient's arm at the biceps. The patient's arm hangs with the elbow bent. The examiner taps the back of the patient's arm just above the elbow with the percussion hammer, feeling for the muscle to contract.
Knee	The patient sits on a table or bench with his feet off the deck. The examiner taps the patient's knee just below the kneecap, on the tendon. The examiner looks for the contraction of the quadriceps (thigh muscle) and movement of the lower leg.
Ankle	The patient sits as above. The examiner places slight pressure on the patient's toes to stretch the Achilles' tendon, feeling for the toes to contract as the Achilles' tendon shortens (contracts).

www.ingramcontent.com/pod-product-compliance
Lightning Source LLC
Chambersburg PA
CBHW062323220526
45469CB00008B/2604